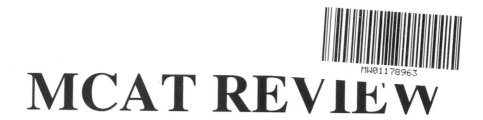

MCAT REVIEW

PEARLS OF WISDOM

Francine,

Thanks for your words of encouragement + support about this book. Good luck always! You will make an awesome pharmacist!

Michael Donnino, M.D.
Paul Tischhauser, Ph.D.
Robert Donnino, M.D.

Copyright © 2002 by Boston Medical Publishing Corporation, Lincoln, NE.

Printed in U.S.A.

The editors would like to extend thanks to Terri Lair for her excellent managing and editorial support.

Art Director: Maryse Charette

This book was produced using Times New Roman and Symbols fonts and computer based graphics with Macintosh® computers

ISBN: 1-58409-052-9

DEDICATION

To Our Parents

Michael Donnino
Robert Donnino

To Karen, Austen and Andrew

Paul Tischhauser

AUTHOR AND EDITOR

Michael Donnino, M.D,
Emergency Medicine/Internal Medicine
Henry Ford Hospital
Detroit, Michigan

AUTHOR: PHYSICS

Paul Tischhauser, Ph.D.
Physicist
Seattle, Washington

ASSOCIATE AUTHOR AND EDITOR

Robert Donnino, M.D.
Internal Medicine
Mount Sinai Hospital
New York, New York

ACKNOWLEDGMENTS

The authors wish to acknowledge, with thanks, the graphic design work of
Dr. Bryce Lord, and the editorial contributions of John McDonagh, Alexandria Muzzin,
Kristine L. Martel, Laura Fiore, and Catherine Donnino.

WE APPRECIATE YOUR COMMENTS!

We appreciate your opinion and encourage you to send us any suggestions or recommendations. Please let us know if you discover any errors, or if there is any way we can make Pearls of Wisdom more helpful to you. We are also interested in recruiting new authors and editors. Please call, write, fax, or e-mail. We look forward to hearing from you.

Send comments to:

**Boston Medical Publishing Corporation
4780 Linden Street, Lincoln, NE, 68516**

**888-MBOARDS (626-2737)
402-484-6118
Fax: 402-484-6552
E-mail: bmp@emedicine.com
www.bmppearls.com**

INTRODUCTION

Congratulations! MCAT Pearls of Wisdom will help you improve your score on the MCAT exam. A few words are appropriate in discussing intent, format, limitations, and use.

Since Pearls is primarily intended as a study aid, the text is written in a rapid-fire question/answer format. This way, readers receive immediate gratification. Questions themselves often contain a "pearl" intended to reinforce the answer. Additional "hooks" may be attached to the answer in various forms including mnemonics, visual imagery, repetition, and humor. Additional information, not requested in the question, may be included in the answer. Emphasis has been placed on distilling trivia and key facts that are easily overlooked and/or quickly forgotten, yet somehow seem to be needed on the MCAT and similar examinations.

Some questions have answers without elaborate explanations. This enhances the ease of reading and rate of learning. Explanations often occur in a later question/answer. Upon reading an answer, the reader may think, "Hm, why is that?" or "Are you sure?" If this happens to you, go check! Truly assimilating these disparate facts into a framework of knowledge absolutely requires further reading of the surrounding concepts. Information learned in response to seeking an answer to a particular question is retained much better than information that is passively learned. Take advantage of this! Use Pearls with your preferred texts handy and open.

Pearls has limitations. We have found some conflicts between sources of information. We have tried to verify in several references the most accurate information. Pearls risks accuracy by aggressively pruning complex concepts down to the simplest kernel – the dynamic knowledge base and practice of the sciences are not like that! Furthermore, new research and practice occasionally deviates from that which likely represents the right answer for test purposes. This text is designed to maximize your score on a test. Refer to your most current sources of information and mentors for further direction.

Pearls is designed to be used, not just read. It is an interactive text. Use a 3 X 5 card and cover the answers – attempt all questions. A study method we recommend is oral, group study, preferably over an extended meal or pitchers. The mechanics of this method are simple and no one ever appears stupid. One person holds Pearls, with answers covered and reads the question. Each person, including the reader, says "check!" when he or she has an answer in mind. After everyone has "checked" in, someone states his/her answer. If this answer is correct, on to the next one; if not, another person says their answer or the answer can be read. Try it, it's ***almost*** fun!

Pearls is also designed to be re-used several times to allow, dare we to use the word, memorization. Two check boxes are provided for any scheme of keeping track of questions answered correctly or incorrectly. Additionally, a "bottom line" section has been provided for each subject area. These sections provide an outline of what we feel is the core material, and can be gone through quickly and efficiently. If you have studied these sections well in advance of the MCAT, they can be easily looked through in a matter of hours as the test nears. Thus, these sections provide a way for the *prepared* student to look over a vast amount of material in a short amount of time (i.e., the week of or before the exam).

We welcome your comments, suggestions, and criticism. Great effort has been made to verify these questions and answers. Some answers may not be the answer you would prefer. Most often this is attributable to variance between original sources. Please make us aware of any errors you find. We hope to make continuous improvements and would greatly appreciate any input with regard to format, organization, content, presentation, or about specific questions. We also are interested in recruiting new contributing authors and publishing new textbooks. Contact our manager at Boston Medical Publishing, Terri Lair, at (toll free) 1-888-MBOARDS. We look forward to hearing from you.

Study hard and good luck!

Michael Donnino

TABLE OF CONTENTS

ORGANIC CHEMISTRY

PHYSICS

THE BOTTOM LINE

BIOLOGY

MOLECULAR BIOLOGY

❑❑ **What is the definition of an enzyme?**

An enzyme is a *protein* (almost always) which serves as a *biological catalyst*.

❑❑ **What is the function of a catalyst in a chemical reaction?**

A catalyst *speeds* the reaction.

❑❑ **How does an enzyme work to speed a reaction?**

The enzyme will *lower the activation energy* needed for a reaction to begin. Remember, a catalyst will *not* change the energy given off or used during the reaction.

❑❑ **Which way will an enzyme speed the following reaction: A <----> B ?**

Since an enzyme simply lowers the activation energy of the reaction, it will increase the reaction rate in both the forward and the reverse directions. Enzymes do not affect the direction in which a reaction will proceed.

❑❑ **What determines the direction in which a reaction will proceed?**

The THERMODYNAMICS of a reaction will determine the direction in which the reaction will proceed. This is discussed further in the general chemistry review. For now, it is important to remember that enzymes are involved with kinetics (speed) and not thermodynamics. Thus,
    KINETICS = SPEED (affected by enzymes)
    THERMODYNAMICS = DIRECTION (not affected by enzymes).

❑❑ **T/F: A catalyst is NOT changed or consumed in a reaction.**

True.

❏❏ **What environmental conditions affect the activity of enzymes?**

Conditions such as temperature, pH, and salt concentration affect the activity of enzymes. Each enzyme has an optimal performance level with reference to each of these parameters.

❏❏ **What is the optimum pH level for most of the enzymes in the human body?**

Most enzymes function optimally at a pH of approximately 7.4, but there are exceptions. For example, some enzymes in the stomach function optimally at a pH of approximately 2 (e.g., pepsin), whereas pancreatic enzymes in the small intestine function optimally at a pH of approximately 8.5.

❏❏ **What happens to an enzyme if its environment becomes too acidic or too alkaline?**

The enzyme can be denatured (i.e., lose its shape) and become inactivated. Very high temperatures can also denature enzymes.

❏❏ **An enzyme is saturated with substrate. What can be done to increase the yield of product?**

Add more enzyme.

❏❏ **Name two types of enzymatic inhibition.**

Competitive and noncompetitive inhibition.

❏❏ **Describe competitive inhibition.**

The inhibitor "competes" with the substrate at the ACTIVE SITE of the enzyme. That is, the inhibitor binds to the enzyme, thus preventing the substrate from attaching at that site. Hence, the reaction is inhibited.

❏❏ **Describe noncompetitive inhibition.**

The inhibitor attaches to an ALLOSTERIC site, which is a location on the enzyme other than the active site. This binding induces a conformational change in the enzyme, which then inhibits the binding of the enzyme to a substrate.
Note: Some substances that bind to allosteric sites are activators, not inhibitors.

❏❏ **What is a zymogen?**

An enzyme that is secreted in an inactive form. For example, pepsinogen is a zymogen. HCl converts pepsinogen to the active form, pepsin.

❑❑ **Which forces are operating in binding of the enzyme/substrate complex?**

Covalent bonds, ionic bonds, hydrogen bonds, and van der Waals forces.

❑❑ **What are the two major types of feedback control that regulate enzyme activity?**

Negative and positive *feedback*.

❑❑ **What differentiates between negative and positive feedback?**

In negative feedback, the product of a sequence of chemical reactions inhibits one of the steps in its synthesis. In *positive* feedback, the product of a chemical reaction activates one of the steps in a sequence of reactions.

❑❑ **Which is more common in the human body, negative or positive feedback?**

Negative feedback is more common.

❑❑ **Name some examples of negative feedback that occur in the human body.**

Some examples of negative feedback in the human body are hormonal control systems and glycolysis. Many more examples exist, making negative feedback the most common mechanism for regulation in the body.

❑❑ **Name some examples of positive feedback.**

Examples of positive feedback include action potentials, childbirth (uterine contractions), and clotting of the blood.

❑❑ **Which type of feedback is involved in the following examples:**

1. **An increase in blood pressure initiates a decrease in renin release by the kidneys. This decrease in renin will serve to lower the blood pressure.**

2. **In digestion, trypsinogen is released from the pancreas. It is then converted to trypsin by enterokinase. The converted trypsin then acts as an enzyme by converting trypsinogen to another molecule of trypsin.**

1- Negative feedback; 2-Positive feedback.

CELLULAR RESPIRATION

❑❑ **What is the overall reaction for cellular respiration?**

$C_6H_{12}O_6 + 6\ O_2 \rightarrow 6\ H_2O + 6\ CO_2 + Energy$

❑❑ **What is the overall reaction for photosynthesis?**

$6\ H_2O + 6\ CO_2 + Energy \rightarrow C_6H_{12}O_6 + 6\ O_2$

❑❑ **What are the three stages of cellular respiration?**

1- Glycolysis
2- Krebs cycle
3- Electron transport chain (ETC)

❑❑ **What is the substrate used in glycolysis?**

Glucose.

❑❑ **How much ATP is invested in glycolysis?**

Two ATP are invested.

❑❑ **How much net ATP is yielded from glycolysis?**

Two ATP are invested, but four are gained. Thus, there is a net gain of two ATP.

❑❑ **What are the products of glycolysis?**

TWO pyruvate molecules.
TWO net ATP molecules.
TWO NADH molecules.

❑❑ **What is the major difference between aerobic and anaerobic respiration?**

Aerobic respiration uses oxygen, whereas anaerobic does not.

❑❑ **What is the fate of pyruvate if *no oxygen* is present (i.e., anaerobic respiration)?**

Pyruvate is converted to lactic acid.

❑❑ **In the conversion of pyruvic acid to lactic acid, what additional substance is produced?**

NADH is *regenerated* into NAD^+. This regeneration is important because NAD^+ may then be used to continue glycolysis.

❑❑ **What is the fate of pyruvate in the presence of oxygen (i.e., in aerobic respiration)?**

In the presence of oxygen, pyruvate is converted to acetyl-CoA and continues through cellular respiration via the Krebs cycle and electron transport chain.

❑❑ **What are two other names for Krebs cycle?**

Tricarboxylic acid cycle and the citric acid cycle.

❑❑ **What is the net ATP produced in anaerobic respiration?**

A net of TWO ATP is produced from glycolysis. Remember, the conversion from pyruvic acid to lactic acid does *not* produce any further ATP. The purpose of this step is to regenerate NAD^+ and to provide a substrate (lactic acid) which can travel through the blood to the liver where it is converted back to glucose (termed the Cori cycle).

❑❑ **What is the total ATP produced in an aerobic reaction?**

The maximum net ATP is 36 (note that some authors will give slightly different numbers).

❑❑ **Where in the eukaryotic cell does glycolysis take place?**

In the cytosol.

❑❑ **Where in the eukaryotic cell does the Krebs cycle take place?**

In the mitochondrion.

❑❑ **Where in the eukaryotic cell does the electron transport chain (ETC) take place?**

In the mitochondrion.

❑❑ **In what specific part of the mitochondrion does the Krebs cycle take place? In what specific part of the mitochondrion does the electron transport chain take place?**

The Krebs cycle takes place in the mitochondrial matrix, whereas the electron transport chain takes place in the inner membrane.

❏❏ **Where does glycolysis take place in bacteria?**

In the cytosol.

❏❏ **Where do the Krebs cycle and the ETC take place in bacteria (prokaryote)?**

In the cell membrane.

❏❏ **Name two differences between bacteria (prokaryotes) and eukaryotes in reference to cellular respiration/ fermentation.**

1- In *bacteria* the Krebs cycle and ETC take place in the *cell membrane*, whereas in eukaryotes these processes take place in the mitochondria.
2- *Bacteria* can use many substances (not just oxygen) as oxidizing agents in respiration, whereas eukaryotes use only oxygen.

❏❏ **Fill in the blanks:**
Glycolysis is a__(how many)__-step process taking place in the __(where)__.
The Krebs cycle is a__(how many)__-step process taking place in the __(where)__ in eukaryotic cells.

Ten, cytosol. *Eight*, mitochondrion.

❏❏ **What happens to the product of glycolysis if it is to be utilized in the Krebs cycle?**

Pyruvate, the product of glycolysis, is transported into the mitochondria. Here the pyruvate is decarboxylated (carbon dioxide is given off) to acetyl-coenzyme A. The acetyl-CoA enters the Krebs cycle.

❏❏ **What does each complete turn of the Krebs cycle generate?**

1 GTP (ATP)
3 NADH
1 FADH$_2$
2 CO$_2$

Note: One molecule of glucose produces two molecules of pyruvate, each of which can be converted to acetyl-CoA and enter the Krebs cycle. Thus, one molecule of glucose would produce twice the number of each of the products listed above.

❏❏ **When pyruvate is reduced to acetyl-CoA, what product is made?**

NADH is produced.

❏❏   **What is the fate of the NADH produced in both glycolysis and the Krebs cycle?**

The NADH enters the electron transport chain and is oxidized. Each NADH generates H^+, which is then used in the process of chemiosmosis to yield approximately 3 ATP.

❏❏   **What is the fate of $FADH_2$?**

The $FADH_2$ enters the electron transport chain and is oxidized. Each $FADH_2$ generates H^+, which is then used in the process of chemiosmosis to yield approximately 2 ATP.

❏❏   **Name the substrates of glycolysis, the Krebs cycle, and the ETC.**

Glycolysis: glucose
Krebs cycle: acetyl-CoA
ETC: NADH, $FADH_2$.

❏❏   **Excess lactic acid may indicate what?**

Lack of oxygen.

❏❏   **What happens to excess lactic acid in the body?**

Excess lactic acid is transported from the tissues to the liver, where it undergoes conversion back into glucose. This cycle is termed the Cori cycle.

❏❏   **What substance will accumulate in a state of decreased blood perfusion to the tissues (i.e., lack of oxygen to the tissues)?**

Lactic acid.

DNA AND PROTEIN SYNTHESIS

❏❏ **What is the basic structure of DNA?**

The basic structure of DNA is called a nucleotide and has three components:
1- NITROGENOUS BASE (adenine, guanine, cytosine, thymine)
2- DEOXYRIBOSE (sugar)
3- PHOSPHATE

❏❏ **How do nucleotides combine to form a strand of DNA?**

These structures are arranged in the classic "double helix" model first elucidated by Watson and Crick. A double helix means that there are two strands of DNA which wind together in a helical fashion.

❏❏ **What are the two categories (i.e., "families") that nitrogenous bases are divided into?**

Purines and pyrimidines.

❑❑   **What is the major structural difference that divides the nitrogenous bases into these two categories?**

Purines are two-ring structures.
Pyrimidines are one-ring structures.

Purine   Pyrimidine

❑❑   **Name the nitrogenous bases that are purines.**

Adenine and guanine.

❑❑   **Name the nitrogenous bases that are pyrimidines.**

Cytosine and thymine in DNA. Cytosine and uracil in RNA.

❑❑   **Which nitrogenous bases pair with each other in DNA?**

Adenine BINDS with thymine (*A-T*).
Guanine BINDS with cytosine (*G-C*).

❑❑   **How does the base pairing differ in RNA?**

Adenine BINDS with *uracil* because there is no thymine in RNA.

❑❑   **Which type of bonds connect paired nitrogenous bases: covalent, ionic, or hydrogen bonds?**

Hydrogen bonds.

❑❑ **How many hydrogen bonds bind guanine with cytosine? Adenine with thymine?**

Guanine-cytosine → 3 hydrogen bonds
Adenine-thymine → 2 hydrogen bonds

Memory tip: To keep in mind that guanine binds cytosine *and* that three hydrogen bonds are used: Gee Cee three.

❑❑ **What is the sequence of the transmission of DNA into a protein?**

(replication)   (transcription)   (translation)

DNA <----------> DNA ------------> RNA -----------> Protein

Note: In recent years, as you know, a new virus called Human Immunodeficiency Virus (HIV) has been elucidated. The HIV virus is a *retro*virus and breaks the traditional sequence by going from RNA to DNA. This is called *reverse* transcription.

Note: Also in recent years a new entity called a prion has been discovered. Prions are proteins that exist in the environment without any RNA or DNA. They are suspected in causing certain diseases including the notorious "Mad Cow Disease."

❑❑ **Where is DNA found?**

In the nucleus.

❑❑ **Where is RNA found?**

RNA is found in the nucleus and/or the cytoplasm.

❑❑ **What is the difference between semi-conservative and conservative processes?**

Conservative means that the two original strands of DNA both remain attached to each other (i.e., they are "conserved"). *Semi-conservative* refers to the fact that each of the two original strands of DNA are separated. Each receives a new complementary strand of DNA, thus forming a DNA molecule with one new and one original strand. Thus, the strands are only partly conserved (hence "semi-conservative").

Conservative: original two DNA strands remain.

Semi-conservative: one of two original DNA strands remains, and one new strand is added.

❑❑ **Is DNA replication semi-conservative or conservative?**

Semi-conservative. When DNA replicates, each parent strand serves as a substrate for the formation of an additional strand. After replication, each parent strand remains with the newly formed strand. Thus, the two original strands are separated.

❑❑ **Is transcription semi-conservative or conservative?**

Conservative. After an RNA molecule is transcribed from the DNA, the two strands of the DNA close, thus maintaining the same two original strands. Thus, this is a conservative process.

❑❑ **Where does DNA replication take place?**

In the nucleus of the cell.

❑❑ **In what direction is new DNA synthesized?**

The new DNA strand is synthesized from the 5' to the 3' direction.

❑❑ **What is the name of the enzymes used to form the new DNA?**

DNA polymerases.

❑❑ **To which end of the DNA strand do DNA polymerases facilitate the addition of new DNA?**

They can add only to the 3' end of the new DNA.

❑❑ **What is needed prior to the action of DNA polymerases, to mark the site of DNA polymerase attachment?**

A primer (short stretch of RNA) is needed to mark the area where the DNA polymerase attaches.

❑❑ **What enzyme is needed to synthesize the primer?**

Primase.

❑❑ **What is the difference between the leading and the lagging strand?**

The leading strand is replicated in a continuous manner from its 5' to 3' end.
The lagging strand is replicated in fragments (called Okazaki fragments) which are synthesized in a 5' to 3' direction, and then attached to each other by DNA ligase to form a continuous strand.

❑❑ **Where does replication begin in prokaryotes?**

At a specific site on the chromosome called the replication origin.

❑❑ **How does this differ from the starting site of DNA replication eukaryotes?**

A: In eukaryotes, DNA replication begins at several different sites along the same chromosome, as opposed to only one replication origin in prokaryotes.

❑❑ **What enzyme is needed to unwind DNA's double helix?**

Helicase.

❑❑ **What is the shape of DNA in prokaryotes?**

Circular.

❑❑ **What is the difference between a exon and an intron?**

A gene is full of many exons and introns. The introns are termed "intervening sequences," as they have no known function and are not translated into proteins. The exons are the portion of the gene that is translated into proteins.
Safety tip: I have noted that students often get these two terms confused. Some mix up the mnemonic "efferent's exit" from the nervous system with exons. Take a second to recognize that "*introns intervene* or *interfere*" and "*EXONS* are *ESSENTIAL*." (Exiting is for the efferent nervous system.)

❑❑ **What are the two steps necessary for protein synthesis from a DNA molecule?**

TRANSCRIPTION (into an RNA molecule), and then TRANSLATION (of the RNA into a protein).

❑❑ **What is the difference between transcription and translation?**

Transcription is conversion of the genetic message from DNA to RNA. *Translation* is conversion of the genetic message from RNA to protein.

❑❑ **What is the enzyme used in transcription?**

RNA polymerase.

❑❑ **Where does transcription take place?**

In the nucleus.

❑❑ **Where does translation take place?**

In the cytoplasm.

❑❑ **Do both transcription and translation take place at the same time in prokaryotes? In eukaryotes?**

In prokaryotes, transcription and translation take place simultaneously. In eukaryotes, transcription takes place first (in the nucleus). Then RNA leaves the nucleus (via nuclear pores) to undergo translation in the cytoplasm.

❑❑ **During which step is protein synthesis regulated?**

Transcription.

❑❑ **In general, how is regulation of protein synthesis performed?**

Specific proteins bind to DNA regulatory sites. These proteins can cause either an increase or a decrease of gene transcription.

❑❑ **What is an operon?**

An operon is a group of genes that code for proteins with associated functions.

❑❑ **What is a codon?**

A codon is a stretch of three amino acids on mRNA.

❑❑ **What does the codon represent or "code" for?**

Each codon of the mRNA represents or "codes" for an amino acid. Though each codon represents only one amino acid, there are sometimes multiple codons for the same amino acid.

❑❑ **What is an anticodon?**

An anticodon is a stretch of three amino acids on tRNA.

❑❑ **What does each tRNA carry?**

An amino acid.

❑❑ **How do codons and anticodons work to form a chain of amino acids (i.e., translation)?**

The anticodon on the tRNA temporarily binds to the complementary codon on the mRNA. Each tRNA is bound to a specific amino acid. The amino acid that is carried by the tRNA is then added to the growing polypeptide chain.

❑❑ **On what structure does translation take place?**

Ribosome.

❑❑ **Where are ribosomes produced?**

In the nucleolus.

❏❏ **What are the three major types of RNA?**

Messenger RNA (mRNA), transfer RNA (tRNA), and ribosomal RNA (rRNA).

❏❏ **What is the product of translation?**

A peptide bond is formed (i.e., a protein).

❏❏ **What is the "A" site?**

"A" stands for aminoacyl-tRNA complex binding site. This is the "incoming site."

❏❏ **What is the "P"site?**

"P" stands for the peptidyl-tRNA binding site. At this site the growing polypeptide is located.

❏❏ **What attaches at the "A" site?**

An incoming aminoacyl-tRNA attaches (i.e., an amino acid attached to tRNA). The anticodon of the tRNA links to the codon of the mRNA.

❏❏ **What happens at the P site?**

The amino acid carried by the tRNA is added to the growing polypeptide chain.

❏❏ **What is translocation?**

The movement of the aminoacyl-tRNA (i.e., an amino acid attached to tRNA) from the A site to the P site.

❏❏ **What is the major difference between the ribosomes of the prokaryotic cell and the eukaryotic cell?**

They differ in the *size* of their subunits:
Ribosomes of the prokaryotic cell are composed of two subunits of sizes 50S and 70S.
Ribosomes of the eukaryotic cell are composed of two subunits of sizes 40S and 60S.

MICROBIOLOGY

❑❑ **What is the definition a virus?**

A virus is often defined as an obligate intracellular parasite composed primarily of RNA or DNA. This means:
"Obligate"= no other options.
 "Intracellular"= must be inside another cell in order to function.
"Parasite"= needs to use another cell's machinery in order to function.

❑❑ **What is the composition of a virus?**

A virus has an RNA or DNA (not both) core surrounded by proteins. This complex is called a nucleocapsid.
Nucleo = RNA, DNA
Capsid = Protein capsule

❑❑ **In addition to the nucleocapsid, a virus may also have an envelope. How is the envelope of the virus obtained?**

The envelope is "stolen" from the cell membrane of the host cell.

❑❑ **Does a virus have intracellular organelles?**

As noted, a virus is an obligate intracellular parasite. As such, the virus depends totally on the host cell for metabolic machinery. Thus, the virus does *not* have any intracellular organelles.

❑❑ **What are examples of "intracellular organelles"?**

Examples of intracellular organelles include mitochondria, Golgi apparatus, endoplasmic reticulum, and lysosomes.

❑❑ **What is a bacteriophage?**

A virus that invades bacteria.

❑❑ **What is an animal virus?**

A virus that infects animal (including human) cells.

❑❑   **How does a bacteriophage invade a host cell?**

The virus binds to the cell membrane and injects its DNA into the host cell. The protein component of the virus does not enter the host cell.

❑❑   **What are the two life cycles of bacteriophages?**

The lytic cycle and the lysogenic cycle.

❑❑   **Briefly describe the lytic cycle.**

Inside the host cell, the virus destroys the host DNA and uses the cell's machinery to replicate its own DNA. Then the host cell lyses (breaks open), and all of the newly replicated viral DNA is released in the form of more bacteriophages.

❑❑   **Briefly describe the lysogenic cycle.**

The viral DNA is integrated into the host cell DNA, and the host cell continues to replicate its own DNA as well as the newly integrated viral DNA (called a prophage). This prophage is then passed on to the host cell's progeny, and may alter the function of these cells. On occasion, the prophage will break loose and undergo viral replication (i.e., enter the lytic cycle).

❑❑   **Briefly describe the life cycle of the animal virus.**

If the virus genome is RNA, it simply uses the cell machinery to replicate itself and to transcribe new viral proteins. Then, new viruses are constructed inside the host cell and can exit the cell without lysing it. Some animal viruses with DNA genomes can integrate into the host DNA to form a provirus, in a manner analogous to the lysogenic cycle.

❑❑   **What is the definition of a prokaryotic cell?**

A single cell *without* a nucleus and *without* any membrane-bound cell organelle or "intracellular organelles." Note that a prokaryotic cell *may* contain ribosomes. Recall that ribosomes are *not* membrane-bound organelles.

❑❑   **In prokaryotic cells, where does glycolysis take place?**

In the cytosol.

❑❑   **In prokaryotic cells, where does the Krebs cycle and the electron transport chain (ETC) take place?**

The plasma membrane.

❑❑   **Name the classic prokaryotic cell.**

BACTERIA!

❑❑ **Match the following: Obligate aerobes, Obligate anaerobes, and/or Facultative anaerobes.**

1- Cannot function in the presence of oxygen.
2- Require oxygen.
3- Will use oxygen if present but can use anaerobic respiration if necessary.

1- Obligate anaerobes.
2- Obligate aerobes.
3- Facultative anaerobes.

❑❑ **What is the difference between a *phototroph* and a *chemotroph*?**

Phototroph: uses light for energy.
Chemotroph: uses chemicals from the environment for energy.

❑❑ **Differentiate between an *autotroph* and a *heterotroph*.**

Autotroph: uses only inorganic carbon dioxide for energy.
Heterotroph: requires at least one organic nutrient like glucose for energy.

❑❑ **The structure of bacteria can be classified as either spherical, spiral, or rod-shaped. What are the scientific names for these shapes?**

Spherical → Cocci
Spiral → Spirochetes
Rod-shaped → Bacilli

❑❑ **What is the difference between Gram-positive bacteria and Gram-negative bacteria?**

Gram-positive bacteria: have a *THICK* layer of PEPTIDOGLYCAN in their cell walls. They have a cell membrane but NO outer membrane.

Gram-negative bacteria: have a *THIN* layer of PEPTIDOGLYCAN. In contrast to Gram-positive bacteria, they have an OUTER membrane in addition to a cell membrane.

❑❑ **How does penicillin destroy bacteria?**

Penicillin disrupts the synthesis of *peptidoglycan.*

❑❑ **Is penicillin more effective against Gram-negative or Gram-positive bacteria? Why?**

Penicillin is more effective at destroying Gram-positive bacteria since they have thick layers of peptidoglycan.

❑❑   **Where do the names Gram-positive and Gram-negative come from?**

From a special laboratory stain developed by Dr. Hans Christian Gram in 1884.

❑❑   **How do bacteria reproduce?**

Binary fission. This means that one parent bacterium divides into two new bacteria.
Thus, <u>exponential growth</u> occurs.

❑❑   **What are the three methods by which bacteria can transfer traits from one to
another?**

1- Conjugation
2- Transformation
3- Transposition

❑❑   **What is conjugation?**

Conjugation is one of three methods that bacteria use to transfer genetic information. In
conjugation, a "male" and a "female" bacterium are connected by pili. Genetic material
is transferred through the pili from one bacterium to the other.

❑❑   **What is transformation?**

Transformation is another method by which bacteria transfer genetic material. In this
method, DNA which are floating around the environment (e.g., from a dead bacterium)
are incorporated into the cell.

❑❑   **What is transposition?**

This is yet another method by which bacteria obtain or transfer genetic material.
Transposition is the transfer of new genetic material into a bacterium by way of a
bacteriophage. A bacteriophage is a virus which infects bacteria. Thus, a virus invades
the bacterium and changes the genetic configuration.

❑❑   **What are the major structural types of fungi?**

Yeasts and molds.

❑❑   **What is the difference between a yeast and a mold?**

Yeast: grow as single cells that reproduce by ASEXUAL BUDDING.
Mold: have hyphae and may reproduce SEXUALLY via SPORES.

❑❑   **Are fungi eukaryotic or prokaryotic cells?**

Eukaryotic cells.

❏❏ **Do fungi have cell walls?**

Yes. The cell wall is made mostly of a substance called chitin.

❏❏ **The cell membrane for eukaryotic cells in humans has cholesterol as a component. What equivalent component do fungi have?**

ERGOSTEROL.

❏❏ **Are fungi obligate aerobes or obligate anaerobes?**

Obligate aerobes.

❏❏ **What do fungi use as a source of carbon?**

All fungi require a preformed organic source of carbon. Thus, most fungi are found in an environment full of decaying matter.

❏❏ **Compare the size of prokaryotes (i.e., bacteria), eukaryotes, and viruses.**

Eukaryotic cell > Prokaryotic cell (bacteria) > Virus.

❏❏ **By what three methods do fungi reproduce?**

1. Budding – A parent cell forms a bud, which grows and eventually breaks away to become an independent daughter cell.
2. Asexual spores – Spores are formed by mitosis from a single fungus.
3. Sexual spores – Two haploid nuclei from two strains of fungi (within the same species) fuse to form a diploid spore. The fungi communicate through fusion of hyphae between the two organisms.

THE EUKARYOTIC CELL

❏❏ **Describe the structure of the nucleus.**

The nucleus is a large, membrane-bound organelle that contains the chromosomes and is surrounded by a nuclear envelope.

❏❏ **What is a nuclear envelope?**

A double membrane with nuclear pores that surrounds the nucleus.

❏❏ **What is the function of nuclear pores?**

These tiny holes allow for the exchange of molecules between the nucleus and the cytoplasm.

❏❏ **What is the nucleolus?**

A dense body of genetic material encoding for rRNA, found within the nucleus.

❏❏ **Describe the two membranes of mitochondria.**

Inner membrane – highly-folded (folds = cristae) membrane. Site of electron transport chain.

Outer membrane – smooth membrane separated from inner membrane by intermembrane space.

❏❏ **What is the matrix of a mitochondrion?**

The compartment surrounded by the inner membrane. Site of Krebs cycle.

❏❏ **What is meant by the description of mitochondria as semi-autonomous?**

Mitochondria contain their own DNA and ribosomes. Despite carrying their own DNA, they still depend on the cell for additional protein synthesis. Thus, they are "semi" autonomous.

❏❏ **What is a lysosome?**

A sac-like, membrane-bound organelle that stores hydrolytic enzymes used for food digestion as well as destruction of damaged organelles. These cells function at an acidic pH of approximately 5.

❑❑ **What is the Golgi apparatus?**

A membranous structure which is involved in packaging, modifying, and distributing secretory products.

❑❑ **Briefly describe the two types of endoplasmic reticulum (ER).**

Rough ER: Intracellular membrane that serves as the site of ribosome attachment. Involved in manufacturing and transporting proteins.

Smooth ER: Intracellular membrane involved in lipid metabolism and the detoxification of some drugs.

❑❑ **Which organ contains a large amount of smooth endoplasmic reticulum?**

Liver. The liver plays a large role in detoxification.

❑❑ **What is the structure of the plasma membrane?**

The plasma membrane is made up of two layers of phospholipids. The hydrophilic head of each phospholipid faces the exterior, while the hydrophobic tail faces the interior. Proteins are integrated throughout the membrane in various arrangements (some on the outside, some partially embedded, some spanning the entire width of the membrane, etc.).

❑❑ **What determines the location of particular amino acids (i.e., protein) in the plasma membrane?**

The charge of the amino acid determines location. The negatively-charged amino acids tend to be located toward the exterior since they are attracted to the hydrophilic head of the phospholipid. The uncharged amino acids tend to be located toward the interior since they are attracted to the hydrophobic (uncharged) tails of the phospholipid.

❑❑ **What is this model of plasma membrane structure called?**

Fluid mosaic model.

❑❑ **What are the types of transport that take place across the plasma membrane?**

Passive transport (e.g., simple diffusion, facilitated diffusion)
Active transport
Endocytosis/Exocytosis

❑❑ **What is osmosis?**

The passive (i.e., requiring no energy) movement of water down its concentration gradient. Water flows from the area of lowest particle concentration to the area of highest particle concentration.

❏❏ **A diabetic patient presents to the emergency department with very high blood sugar and a blood osmolarity of 500 mosm. How would body cells be affected by this osmolarity? Hint: The approximate osmolarity of a cell is 300 mosm.**

Fluid from the cell would flow into the bloodstream because of the higher osmolarity in that location. Body cells would shrink because of the loss of fluid. Remember, water flows to the area of highest particle concentration (i.e., highest osmolarity). This fluid shift explains why diabetics have to urinate often and are dehydrated when they present to emergency departments with very high blood sugar levels.

❏❏ **What is facilitated diffusion?**

Facilitated diffusion is a type of passive transport (i.e., requires no energy) in which a molecule is "carried" across the plasma membrane (down its concentration gradient) by a carrier protein.

❏❏ **How does active transport differ from facilitated diffusion?**

Active transport requires energy to move molecules typically against a concentration gradient. Facilitated diffusion requires no energy, and molecules move down the concentration gradient.

❏❏ **What is secondary active transport?**

One molecule (such as sodium) is *actively* pumped out of the cell and creates a concentration gradient. The return of the molecule (e.g., sodium) is coupled with a *passive* co-transport of another molecule (e.g., glucose). Thus, glucose exhibits secondary active transport.

❏❏ **What is endocytosis? Exocytosis?**

In endocytosis, a portion of the plasma membrane invaginates and pinches off from the rest of the membrane, forming a vesicle around the entering molecule. In exocytosis, a vesicle inside the cell fuses with the plasma membrane, releasing the contents outside the cell.

❏❏ **What complex in the plasma membrane is largely responsible for creating and maintaining the electrochemical gradient across the membrane?**

The sodium-potassium pump, which pumps sodium out of the cell and potassium into the cell.

❏❏ **What type of transport does the sodium-potassium pump use?**

Active transport (ATP is used for energy).

❑❑ **How many sodium molecules are pumped into a cell per potassium molecules pumped out of a cell?**

Three sodium molecules are pumped in for every two potassium molecules that are pumped out.

❑❑ **What is a plasma membrane receptor?**

A protein in the plasma membrane that binds to a specific molecule (e.g., a hormone; a neurotransmitter).

❑❑ **What are the 3 major components of the cytoskeleton?**

1- Microtubules (composed of tubulin)
2- Microfilaments (composed of actin)
3- Intermediate filaments (varied composition)

❑❑ **What are the structural components of cilia and flagella in the eukaryotic cell?**

Both cilia and flagella contain a cytoplasmic matrix with nine sets of associated microtubules and a basal body to anchor the structures to the cell membrane.

❑❑ **What is the function of cilia and flagella?**

They are most often used for movement of the cell, or to move small particles and fluids across the cell surface.

❑❑ **What is the difference between cilia and flagella?**

There is little difference between these terms. Flagella tend to be longer than cilia, and cells usually have only one or a few flagella compared to multiple cilia.

CIRCULATORY SYSTEM

❑❑ **List some of the functions of the circulatory system.**

Delivery of oxygen and nutrients.
Removal of metabolic waste products.
Transport of regulatory molecules (e.g., hormones).
Transport of chemicals and enzymes.
Transport of molecules and cells essential to the immune system.
Thermoregulation.

❑❑ **What is the "pacemaker" of the heart?**

The *sinoatrial node* (SA node). This is located in the right atrium and paces the heart at a rate of 60-100 beats per minute.

❑❑ **Which division of the autonomic nervous system (sympathetic or parasympathetic) slows down the heart?**

Parasympathetic nervous system. More specifically, cranial nerve number X (vagus nerve) innervates the heart and slows it down.

Note: I do not think you will need to know the 12 cranial nerves for the MCAT exam, but you should be familiar with cranial nerve number X (vagus nerve). It also innervates most of the viscera (i.e., internal organs).

❑❑ **Do arteries transport oxygenated or deoxygenated blood?**

This is a trick question as arteries transport both. Arteries are named only by the fact that they transport blood *away* from the heart. While most arteries carry oxygenated blood to the tissues, the pulmonary artery transports deoxygenated blood to the lungs.

Tip: Artery = Away

❑❑ **Name the chambers of the heart.**

Right atrium, right ventricle, left atrium, left ventricle.

❑❑ **Starting with the right atrium, trace the flow of blood through the body.**

Right atrium → Right ventricle → Pulmonary artery → Lungs → Pulmonary veins → Left atrium → Left ventricle → Aorta → Body (tissues) → Superior/Inferior vena cava → Right atrium.

❑❑ **What are some of the differences between the atria and the ventricles?**

The atria are located above the ventricles and receive blood from the body (right atrium) and the lungs (left atrium). Blood then drains into the ventricles where it is pumped to the body (left ventricle) and the lungs (right ventricle). Since the ventricles function to pump blood out of the heart, they are stronger and larger than the atria.

❑❑ **What is the aorta?**

The aorta is the largest artery in the body. Blood from the left ventricle is pumped into the aorta and travels to the tissues through smaller arteries branching off of the aorta .

❑❑ **What are the superior/inferior vena cava?**

The superior and inferior vena cava are the largest veins in the body. Blood from the tissues is returned to the right atrium via the superior and inferior vena cava.

❑❑ **Starting with an artery, trace the flow of blood through the vasculature of the body.**

Artery → Arterioles → Capillaries → Venules → Veins.

❑❑ **Which vascular structure has the most control over blood pressure?**

The *arterioles* have the most control over blood pressure. The sympathetic nervous system innervates the smooth muscle in the arterioles and causes vasoconstriction. The vasoconstriction results in an increase in blood pressure.

❑❑ **In which vascular structure does the exchange of gases with the lung take place?**

Capillaries.

❑❑ **How does gas exchange take place between the capillaries and the alveoli of the lung?**

Gas is exchanged by simple diffusion.

❑❑ **Associate the following with either artery or vein:**
1- **Muscular, strong structure**
2- **Bright red blood**
3- **Dark red blood**
4- **Pulsating, brisk bleeding**
5- **High pressure system**
6- **Slow, sluggish bleeding**
7- **Low pressure system**

1-Artery, 2-Artery, 3-Vein, 4-Artery, 5-Artery, 6-Vein, 7-Vein

❏❏ **Which branch of the autonomic nervous system constricts the arterioles, thus raising blood pressure?**

The sympathetic nervous system causes constriction of the arterioles (i.e., vasoconstriction).

❏❏ **Which branch of the autonomic nervous system dilates the arterioles, causing relaxation and thus decreased blood pressure?**

This is a trick question! The only branch of the autonomic nervous system that innervates blood vessels is the sympathetic nervous system. The sympathetic nervous system maintains a baseline constriction on the blood vessels. If pressure needs to be increased, the sympathetic nervous system causes increased vasoconstriction. If pressure needs to be decreased, the lack of sympathetic stimulation causes decreased vasoconstriction (i.e., vasodilation).

❏❏ **How does the circulatory system aid in thermoregulation?**

When the body is overheated, the blood vessels dilate so that heat is lost through the skin. When the body is trying to conserve heat, the peripheral arteries vasoconstrict to prevent loss of heat through the skin.

❏❏ **What is the difference between systole and diastole?**

Systole: contraction phase of the heart.
Diastole: relaxation phase of the heart.

Note: Systole and diastole can further be broken down into atrial systole and ventricular systole as well as atrial and ventricular diastole.

❏❏ **Which is higher, the pressure of blood in the arteries during systole or during diastole?**

The blood pressure is higher during systole because that is when the left ventricle is contracting and pushing blood through the arteries. Typically, a person's blood pressure is reported as two values—one for systole and one for diastole. For example, if a person has a blood pressure of "120 over 80," the 120 refers to the arterial blood pressure during systole, and the 80 refers to the arterial blood pressure during diastole.

❏❏ **What is cardiac output?**

Cardiac output = heart rate x stroke volume (volume of blood pumped out of the left ventricle per contraction).

❑❑ **How many liters of blood does the average human body contain?**

4-6 liters.

❑❑ **What is the composition of the blood?**

The blood is composed of *plasma* (55%) and *cells* (45%). The plasma includes water, salts, ions, proteins, and other substances. Cells (or formed elements) include red blood cells (erythrocytes), white blood cells (leukocytes), and platelets.

❑❑ **What are the basic functions of each of these formed elements: erythrocytes, leukocytes, and platelets?**

Red blood cells (erythrocytes):   Transport oxygen to the tissues. They also help transport carbon dioxide back to the lungs (minor role).
White blood cells (leukocytes): Provide defense (immune system) for the body.
Platelets (thrombocytes):   Involved with blood clotting.

❑❑ **A patient presents to the emergency department with a fever and productive cough. He is ultimately diagnosed with pneumonia. A blood test measures the white blood cell count. Do you expect this will be low, normal, or high?**

High. Infection generally causes an increased production of white blood cells for defense.

❑❑ **What are the three *structural* differences between adult and fetal circulation?**

The fetus has three structures that the normal adult does not have:
1- Ductus venosus (liver bypass).
2- Foramen ovale (opening from right to left atrium).
3- Ductus arteriosus (lung bypass; duct from pulmonary artery to aorta).

❑❑ **What is the physiologic purpose of the three structural modifications of fetal circulation?**

During fetal life, the lungs and liver are essentially non-functional. On the other hand, a large amount of blood needs to be circulated through the placenta to the tissues. These modifications allow for oxygenated blood (entering through the umbilical vein) to bypass the liver (through the ductus venosus) and the lungs (through the foramen ovale) and travel to the tissues. Deoxygenated blood returns through the right atrium to the pulmonary artery and bypasses the lungs (through the ductus arteriosus) on its return to the placenta via the two umbilical arteries.

❑❑ **What is the substance contained in red blood cells that transports oxygen?**

Hemoglobin.

❑❑ **What portion of the hemoglobin molecule binds oxygen?**

Hemoglobin consists of a protein portion and a heme portion. The heme portion contains an iron molecule that binds oxygen.

❑❑ **How many oxygen molecules can be bound by one hemoglobin molecule?**

Four.

❑❑ **What does "cooperative binding" mean?**

Cooperative binding means that the binding of one oxygen molecule increases the tendency for the binding of a second oxygen molecule. The same principle applies for the third and fourth oxygen molecules.

❑❑ **What are the four blood types?**

Type A, Type B, Type AB, and Type O.

❑❑ **What is the lymphatic system?**

The lymphatic system is an accessory drainage system for the blood. About 1% of blood is leaked from capillaries into the interstitial space. The lymphatic system drains this runoff and delivers it back into the blood in the upper chest. Perhaps the most important aspect of this drainage is removing large proteins from the interstitial space. The lymphatic system also plays an essential role in transporting lipids from the digestive system.

❑❑ **You are at a wedding and suddenly one of the young groomsmen passes out. What is a possible mechanism for this? Hint: What mechanism facilitates blood return to the heart?**

The venous system returns blood to the heart. The venous system is a low-pressure system. Thus, blood is returned to the heart by skeletal muscle "pumping." That is, the contraction of skeletal muscles squeezes the veins and "pumps" blood back to the right atrium. Thus, standing "at attention" for a long period of time without moving the legs/bending at the knees does not allow for the skeletal muscle pump to return blood to the heart. Ultimately, the heart cannot effectively pump blood to the brain and the groomsman hits the carpet.

❑❑ **What is the blood type of the universal donor?**

O.

❑❑ **What is the blood type of the universal recipient?**

AB.

❏❏ **Why is type O blood considered the universal donor?**

Type O blood contains neither A nor B antigens. If type O blood is donated to a
recipient, an adverse reaction is unlikely since no A or B antigens are present. Note that
both A and B antibodies *are* present and will react with antigens from type A, type B, or
type AB blood donors. Thus, people with type O blood are poor recipients.

❏❏ **Why is type AB blood considered to be the universal recipient?**

People with type AB blood form both A and B antigens and therefore no A or B
antibodies. Thus, they may receive any of the other blood types without much risk for an
adverse reaction.

❏❏ **What is the difference between Rh-negative and Rh-positive blood?**

A person may have either an Rh-positive or an Rh-negative blood type. This is
determined by the presence (positive) or absence (negative) of an antigen termed the Rh
factor.

❏❏ **A pregnant mother has Rh-negative blood and the father has Rh-positive
blood. Can this harm the fetus? Why or why not?**

Yes. If the fetus has inherited the Rh-factor from the father (i.e., Rh-positive blood) then
the mother may make antibodies to this factor. Those antibodies may then cross into the
fetus and attack the child's red blood cells. Note that this takes place typically on a
second rather than first pregnancy. The mother's immune system needs to be "primed"
first.

IMMUNE SYSTEM

❑❑ **What is the definition of an antigen?**

Any substance that the immune system recognizes as foreign.

❑❑ **What are the two general categories of immune system response?**

1- Non-specific.
2- Specific.

❑❑ **What does the "specific" immune system response refer to?**

The term "specific" is used because the immune system "recognizes" the "specific" antigen and responds with cells directed at that particular antigen. This is in contrast to the non-specific immune system response that defends against all antigens without identifying them.

❑❑ **The non-specific immune system can be divided into external and internal defenses. What are some external defenses?**

Protection by skin and mucous membranes.

❑❑ **What are some examples of internal non-specific defenses?**

Inflammatory response: mediated by substances (i.e., histamine and others) from *mast* cells and basophils. The inflammatory response brings "troops for battle"/ heals wounds.

Phagocytosis: antigens engulfed indiscriminately by neutrophils, monocytes, macrophages, and eosinophils.

Mucociliary pump: Cilia in the respiratory tract mechanically brush away foreign particles.

❑❑ **What are the two major divisions of the *specific* immune system?**

1- Cell-mediated immunity.
2- Humoral immunity.

❑❑ **What type of cells mediate the cell-mediated immune system?**

T lymphocytes.

❑❑   **What type of cells mediate the humoral response?**

B lymphocytes.

❑❑   **Where does the word "humoral" come from?**

The word humoral comes from the word "humors" which was used to describe what we now call blood. The humoral system thus received its name because of its role in defending against *bloodborne invaders*.

❑❑   **What are the differences between the cell-mediated and humoral responses?**

The *humoral* immune system defends the body mainly against extracellular bacteria and viruses in the blood. B lymphocytes differentiate into plasma cells that secrete antibodies. These antibodies bind to and neutralize invading microbes. These antibodies are produced to specifically attack a given antigen.

The *cell-mediated* immune system defends the body mainly against intracellular bacteria, viruses inside cells, fungi, and tumors. T lymphocytes are the mediators of this system and they do not secrete antibodies. The name "cell-mediated" is derived from the fact that the T lymphocyte, or the "cell," directly confronts invaders and no antibodies are involved. T lymphocytes are adept at recognizing cells that have been invaded by foreign microbes.

❑❑   **Name the five different types of immunoglobulins.**

IgM, IgG, IgA, IgE, and IgD.

❑❑   **Label the following immunoglobulins with the correct description:**

IgM IgG IgA IgE IgD

1- **Contained in secretions like mucous and breast milk**
2- **Involved in hypersensitivity or allergic reactions**
3- **Most abundant**
4- **Likely involved in antigen recognition**
5- **First to respond to incoming antigens**

1-IgA, 2-IgE, 3-IgG, 4-IgD, 5-IgM.

❑❑   **What is complement? How does it aid in defense?**

Complement is a term for a group of proteins that combine together to form a *membrane attack complex*.   The membrane attack complex seeks out and destroys infected cells. Complement may destroy antigens that have already been bound by antibodies. Thus, these proteins "complement" the rest of the defense systems.

❑❑ **What is the difference between T cell independent and T cell dependent response?**

Most antigens that invade our bodies are "swallowed" by a phagocytic cell, usually a macrophage. This cell then presents a portion of the antigen to a helper T cell. The helper T cell then calls for cytotoxic T cells (cell-mediated response) and for B cells (humoral response). Thus, the B cells are dependent on helper T cells in this scenario. The other possible scenario is that a B cell directly confronts an antigen in the blood and a response is elicited. This would be a T cell independent response.

❑❑ **Which would be more apt (cell-mediated or humoral) in fighting the following?**

1- Viruses
2- Intracellular bacteria
3- Extracellular bacteria
4- Fungi

Extracellular bacteria are best fought with the humoral immune system. Viruses, intracellular bacteria, and fungi are best fought with the cell-mediated immune system.

❑❑ **What is the cellular defect caused by the Acquired Immunodeficiency Syndrome (AIDS)?**

Defective helper T cells (caused by the HIV virus).

❑❑ **What types of infections are prevalent in patients with AIDS?**

Keeping in mind that AIDS is a defect in T cells (i.e., cell-mediated immunity), some common manifestations include fungal infections (e.g., candida in the mouth, and others), viruses, and intracellular bacterial infections (e.g., tuberculosis).

❑❑ **If a patient has a disease that causes deficiency in B cells, such as Bruton's agammaglobulinemia, what types of infections would be expected?**

Bacterial infections (extracellular).

❑❑ **Where do B cells and T cells originate? Where do they mature?**

All blood cells (red and white) *originate* in the *bone marrow*. Thus, both B and T cells (which are white blood cells) originate in the bone marrow. B lymphocytes mature in the bone marrow but T cells do not. T cells migrate to the thymus for maturation.

Memory tip: B lymphocytes mature in the Bone marrow.
              T lymphocytes mature in the Thymus.

❑❑ **How did "T" lymphocyte get its name?**

"T" was named after thymus since T lymphocytes mature there.

❏❏ **How did "B lymphocyte" get its name?**

B lymphocytes were *not* named for the bone marrow where they mature, although this is certainly convenient for MCAT studying. Actually, the B lymphocyte is named after the bursa of Fabricius, which is where B cells mature in birds. The B lymphocyte was first identified in the bursa of Fabricius of chickens.

❏❏ **What are some storage sites of lymphocytes throughout the body?**

Spleen : Serves to filter the blood by removing antigens and old or defective red blood cells from circulation.

Lymph nodes: Also act to filter out antigens and dead cells from the lymph before the lymph enters the bloodstream. They are often enlarged and palpable during infection.

❏❏ **What is the difference between primary and secondary response?**

A primary response develops when an antigen is encountered for the first time. The immune system is "taken by surprise" and is slower to respond to this initial attack. Thus, a typical response takes about 7-10 days.
A secondary response develops when an antigen is encountered for a second (or more) time. The immune system is "ready" for the antigen this time, and the response is much faster.

❏❏ **Bonus (will not be tested): Who first noticed the phenomena of primary and secondary response?**

Over 2400 years ago, Thucydides (the Greek historian) noted that plague victims were being cared for by others who had previously been infected but survived. The care-givers did not develop the disease a second time because, as we now know, the immune system response was swifter and more effective on subsequent exposures.

❏❏ **What is the fate of an antigen when bound by an antibody?**

The antigen-antibody complex will be destroyed by one of three mechanisms:
1. Engulfed by macrophages (i.e., phagocytosis).
2. Destroyed by special lymphocytes (e.g., natural killer cells).
3. Destroyed by complement proteins.

RESPIRATORY SYSTEM

❑❑ **Place the following structures in the correct order in which air travels into the lungs:**
Alveoli Bronchi Mouth (Oral Cavity) Bronchioles Pharynx Larynx Trachea

Oral Cavity→Pharynx→Larynx→Trachea→Bronchi→Bronchioles→Alveoli.

❑❑ **Which structure of the respiratory system contains smooth muscle, is innervated by the autonomic nervous system, and controls airflow via constriction and dilatation?**

Bronchioles.

❑❑ **Which structure of the respiratory system is directly involved in gas exchange?**

Alveoli.

❑❑ **What is surfactant? How does it function?**

Surfactant is a lipid that forms a thin layer coating each alveolus. Surfactant serves to lower the surface tension of the alveoli and facilitate gas exchange across the membranes.

❑❑ **How are oxygen and carbon dioxide exchanged in the respiratory system?**

Oxygen and carbon dioxide are exchanged between the alveoli of the lung and the capillaries of the vascular system by *simple diffusion*.

❑❑ **What is the primary muscle involved in breathing?**

The diaphragm.

❑❑ **Is inspiration an active or passive process? Explain the process.**

Inspiration is an active process. The process begins with the contraction of the diaphragm and sometimes the intercostal muscles. This contraction increases the volume in the chest cavity. A negative pressure differential is created (relative to the external environment), thus favoring the flow of air from the environment into the lungs. The air (about 70% nitrogen, 21% oxygen, and 9% other gases) rushes down the pressure gradient and into the lungs.

❏❏   **Is expiration an active or passive process?**

Under normal respiratory conditions, expiration is a passive process, which occurs with the relaxation of the rib cage and the diaphragm. In situations where additional ventilation is needed (e.g., during an asthma attack or during exercise), expiration can have an active component. In this situation the intercostal muscles can actively force air out of the lungs.

❏❏   **What is the function of hemoglobin?**

To bind and release (i.e., carry and drop off) oxygen.

❏❏   **How many subunits compose each molecule of hemoglobin?**

Four.

❏❏   **How many oxygen molecules can bind to one hemoglobin molecule?**

Four oxygen bind to one hemoglobin molecule.

❏❏   **What is the "oxygen-hemoglobin dissociation curve"?**

This curve describes the partial pressures of oxygen (x-axis) and the percent saturation of hemoglobin (y-axis).

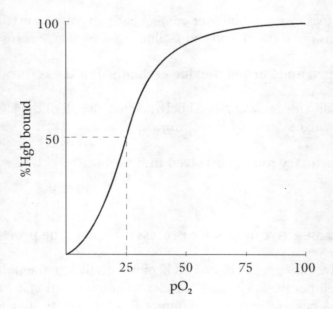

❏❏   **What is p50?**

The partial pressure of oxygen that is required to saturate exactly 50% of hemoglobin.

❑❑ **When the curve shifts to the right, does the p50 increase or decrease?**

Increase.

❑❑ **What causes the curve to shift to the right?**

Increase in temperature, decreased pH, increased CO_2, or increased 2,3 DPG.

❑❑ **What causes the curve shift to the left?**

Decrease in temperature, increased pH, or decreased CO_2. Carbon monoxide poisoning can also shift the curve to the left.

❑❑ **What are two functions of the respiratory system other than gas exchange?**

1- *Thermoregulation*: Increased ventilation dissipates heat and could be considered a "cooling method" (seen in animals [e.g., panting dog] but not typically in humans).

2- *Immunity* (protect against disease): The respiratory tract contains the mucociliary pump, which serves to brush bacteria upward and out of the respiratory tract. In addition, an immunoglobulin (IgA) is secreted in the respiratory tract to protect against invading bacteria. Alveolar macrophages which also serve to defend against bacteria are also stationed here (see "Immune System" for further information).

DIGESTIVE SYSTEM

❑❑ **Digestion of which substances begins in the oral cavity?**

Digestion of *polysaccharides* begins in the oral cavity by salivary amylase. Remember that the digestion of proteins and lipids does *not* begin here. Also note that in the oral cavity, saliva moistens and lubricates food to prepare for digestion.

❑❑ **The stomach secretes "gastric juice." What is the function of this gastric juice?**

Gastric juice:
- KILLS bacteria.
- Disrupts intercellular connections of substances being digested.
- Converts *pepsinogen to pepsin*.
- Maintains a low pH (about 2). This is necessary for pepsin activity.
- Reduces food to a "nutrient broth" (i.e., chyme).

❑❑ **What is the function of pepsin?**

To digest proteins. Remember that in the stomach the digestion of polysaccharides and lipids does *not* take place. The salivary amylase which begins the digestion of polysaccharides in the oral cavity is rendered inactive by the high acidity of the stomach.

❑❑ **What is the function of the small intestine?**

Digestion and absorption. Digestion of proteins, polysaccharides, and lipids occurs here. The small intestine has the *largest surface area* of the digestive tract. Thus, most of the food and nutrients are absorbed here.

❑❑ **What are the breakdown products of proteins, lipids, and polysaccharides?**

Proteins → amino acids.
Lipids → fatty acid and glycerol.
Polysaccharides → monosaccharides.

❑❑ **After proteins and polysaccharides are broken down into their derivative components, how are they incorporated into the body?**

After breakdown, they are absorbed into *capillaries* and into the venous system. The veins transport the blood to the liver and then into the right atrium for circulation to the tissues.

❑❑   **After lipids are broken down into fatty acids and glycerol, how are they incorporated into the body?**

They are absorbed into *lacteals* that lead to the lymphatic system.

❑❑   **Which of the following has the largest surface area?**
Stomach   Small intestine
Esophagus   Large intestine
Rectum

Small intestine.

❑❑   **What structures increase the surface area of the small intestine?**

Villi, microvilli, and brush border allow for the increased surface area.

❑❑   **Which glands produce digestive secretions that are transported to the small intestine?**

Pancreas and liver.

❑❑   **What digestive substance is produced in the liver?**

Bile. The liver secretes bile into ducts that lead to the gallbladder. Bile is then stored in the gallbladder until needed for digestion. When needed for digestion, the gallbladder secretes bile into ducts that lead to the small intestine.

❑❑   **What is the function of bile?**

Bile aids in the absorption of fats (emulsifies lipids).

❑❑   **What does the pancreas contribute to the digestive tract?**

The pancreas secretes the following into the small intestine:
1- Hydrolytic enzymes (i.e., amylase, lipase, etc.)
2- Bicarbonate: This is a basic substance that functions to neutralize the acidic stomach secretions.

❑❑   **What is the function of the large intestine?**

By the time food has reached the large intestine, the bulk of the absorption has already occurred. Although some absorption of nutrients continues, the major function of the large intestine is the formation of stool by reabsorption of sodium, water and other ions. The large intestine leads to the ano-rectal canal and to the anus, where excretion takes place.

❑❑ **Which branch of the nervous system stimulates digestion?**

The parasympathetic nervous system stimulates digestion. Note that an enteric (intestinal) nervous system also exists.

❑❑ **How is food pushed along through the digestive system?**

Peristalsis consists of coordinated contractions of smooth muscle, which squeeze food along the digestive tract. This passage of food is also regulated by sphincters, which open to allow food to pass through.

KIDNEY

❑❑ **What are the functions of the kidney?**

Regulate salt and water.
Regulate blood pressure and volume.
Maintain acid/base balance.
Stimulate growth of red blood cells (RBCs).

❑❑ **What substances are secreted by the kidney? What are their functions?**

1- Erythropoietin: Stimulates development of red blood cells in the bone marrow.
2- Renin: Helps in maintaining blood pressure and volume through the angiotensin pathway.

❑❑ **Briefly describe the gross anatomy of the kidney.**

Within the kidney, urine is produced in the cortex (outer layer) and the medulla (inside the cortex). Urine is emptied into the renal pyramids (interior to the medulla) and then the renal pelvis (innermost region of the kidney) before finally leaving the kidney through the ureter.

❑❑ **Trace the passage of filtrate from the blood passing through a nephron into the renal pelvis.**

Filtrate from the blood leaves the capillaries at the glomerulus and is collected in Bowman's capsule which surrounds the glomerular capillaries. The filtrate then enters the proximal convoluted tubule and continues through the loop of Henle. Finally, the filtrate passes through the distal convoluted tubule, then through the collecting duct and out into the renal pelvis.

❑❑ **What are the three ways that the kidney regulates the passage of solute?**

1- Filtration.
2- Reabsorption.
3- Secretion.

❑❑ **How does the kidney contribute to the regulation of osmolarity?**

Osmoreceptor cells in the hypothalamus monitor the osmolarity of the blood. If the blood is hyperosmotic, then ADH (antidiuretic hormone) is released from the posterior pituitary gland. (Recall: ADH is produced by the hypothalamus and stored in the posterior pituitary.) ADH then acts on the distal tubule and collecting duct of the kidney to *reabsorb water and urea*. The reabsorption of water dilutes the blood, thus lowering the osmolarity.

Also note: Hyperosmotic fluid which passes through the hypothalamus also causes *THIRST*. Thus, we drink additional fluid, dilute the blood, and cause a decrease in osmolarity.

❑❑ **Where are wastes from the kidney stored before excretion? How do they arrive at this location?**

Bladder. Waste (urine) from the kidney flows to the bladder via ureters. From the bladder, urine is EXCRETED via the urethra. Kidney→ureter→bladder→urethra.

❑❑ **What is the structural part of the nephron whose longer length would allow for increased concentration ability of the kidney?**

The loop of Henle.

❑❑ **What two hormones act on the kidney? What do they do?**

Aldosterone: Steroid that acts at distal tubule to *reabsorb sodium* and secrete potassium. This leads to reabsorption of water.

Vasopressin (or antidiuretic hormone "ADH"): Protein that acts at the collecting duct to reabsorb *water and urea*.

MUSCLE AND SKELETAL SYSTEM

❑❑ **What are the three different types of muscles?**

Skeletal, cardiac, and smooth muscle.

❑❑ **Compare and contrast the three types of muscles.**

Types of Muscle

	SKELETAL	SMOOTH	CARDIAC
Structure	Striations	No striations	Striations and intercalated discs
Nervous system innervation	Somatic	Autonomic	Myogenic with autonomic modification
Voluntary or involuntary	Generally voluntary	Generally involuntary	Generally involuntary
Location	Attached to bones of both axial and appendicular skeleton	Digestive tract, reproductive tract, vasculature (mostly arteries/arterioles)	Heart
Components	Troponin/ tropomyosin	No troponin	Troponin/ tropomyosin

❏❏ **What branch of the nervous system innervates (stimulates) skeletal muscle?**

The somatic nervous system.

❏❏ **What branch of the nervous system stimulates cardiac and smooth muscle?**

The autonomic nervous system.

❏❏ **Describe the structure of a sarcomere.**

A sarcomere is made up of thin and thick filaments arranged in a specific configuration. A single sarcomere extends from one so-called Z line to another Z line. Within each sarcomere there is an "I band" which is an area of only thin filaments, an H zone which is an area with only thick filaments, and an "A band" which is a region where the thick and thin filaments overlap.

❏❏ **I am an ion who rushes into muscle cells. I cause contraction of smooth, skeletal, and cardiac muscle although I use different mechanisms in each of these cells. Who am I?**

Calcium.

❏❏ **How does the calcium contribute to contraction in skeletal muscle?**

Calcium is released from T-tubules after stimulation from acetylcholine (neurotransmitter for the somatic nervous system). The calcium then binds to troponin. The troponin-calcium binding causes tropomyosin to be "opened" for attachment of myosin (see below). Myosin and actin then link and cause muscle contraction.

❏❏ **What type of muscle is considered involuntary? Voluntary?**

Skeletal muscle is usually "voluntary", whereas smooth and cardiac muscle are typically "involuntary." Exceptions to this do exist but they are rare. For instance, a Buddhist monk may be able to "voluntarily" reduce his heart rate (cardiac muscle) to 10 beats/minute. Or, a reflex hammer can elicit an "involuntary" contraction of skeletal muscle. Despite these exceptions, the MCAT exam will most likely test the general rule that skeletal muscle is voluntary, whereas smooth and cardiac are involuntary.

❏❏ **What is rigor mortis? What is the cause of this on a molecular level?**

RIGOR MORTIS is the term for a stiffening of the body which takes place after death. This ultimately occurs because of an inability to return calcium to the sarcoplasmic reticulum. Thus, the actin and myosin bridges stay attached (no ATP to break bonds).

❏❏ **What are the major functions of our skeletal system?**

Protection of the internal organs and structure of the body.

❏❏ **What are the three major types of bone cells? What are their functions?**

Osteoblasts: BUILD bone.
Osteocytes: mature bone cells.
Osteoclasts: RESORB bone (break down).

❏❏ **What is the function of parathyroid hormone? How does it work?**

Parathyroid hormone stimulates osteoclasts to break down bone. This increases calcium in the blood. Thus, parathyroid hormone plays a significant role in the regulation of calcium.

❏❏ **What is the function of calcitonin? How does it work?**

Calcitonin inhibits osteoclasts and thus halts the breakdown of bone. This decreases the calcium in the blood. Calcitonin is not as important in calcium regulation as parathyroid hormone but it does play a role as noted.

❏❏ **What are the three major fiber types that make up connective tissue?**

Collagen fibers: made up of a protein called *collagen* and are notable for their great strength.

Elastic fibers: made up of a protein called *elastin* and are notable for their elasticity.

Reticular fibers: join connective tissues and other tissues.

❏❏ **What is the general difference between loose and dense connective tissue?**

Loose connective tissue is made up of loosely arranged fibers as in bone marrow and the liver. Dense connective tissue is made up of a greater proportion of collagen fibers than loose connective tissue. It is thus stronger than loose connective tissue and makes up ligaments and tendons.

❏❏ **What is the difference between a ligament and a tendon?**

Ligament: connects bone to bone.
Tendon: connects muscle to bone.

❏❏ **What is cartilage?**

It is a special type of dense connective tissue, made up of collagen fibers and a substance called chondrin. Cartilage gives support to structures such as the nose and outer ears.

❏❏ **Name the two types of bone.**

Compact and spongy (cancellous).

ENDOCRINE

❑❑ **What is a hormone?**

A *chemical messenger* that travels via the *blood*.

❑❑ **What is the difference between an endocrine and an exocrine gland?**

An *endocrine* gland is one that releases *hormones* into the blood (*DUCTLESS*).
An *exocrine* gland releases its products (a variety of substances) into *DUCTS*.

❑❑ **What is a duct?**

Generally speaking, a duct is a tube through which secretions or excretions flow.

❑❑ **What is a paracrine cell? Autocrine cell?**

Not all chemical messengers are released into the blood stream or into the ducts. Some just communicate BETWEEN CELLS or WITH THEMSELVES.

PARACRINE: Chemical messenger released from one cell to an *adjacent cell*.

AUTOCRINE: Chemical messenger released from one cell which then *acts on itself*.

❑❑ **Name some examples of <u>ex</u>ocrine glands.**

Examples include:
- Pancreas (releases enzymes into *ducts* which lead to small intestine).
- Liver (releases bile into *ducts* which go to gallbladder for storage).
- Gallbladder (releases stored bile into *ducts* which lead to small intestine).

❑❑ **Name some examples of <u>endo</u>crine glands.**

Examples include:

- Pancreas (releases glucagon and/or insulin into blood to regulate glucose).
- Thyroid (releases thyroid hormone into blood).
- Hypothalamus (releases multiple hormones into blood vessels that lead to the anterior pituitary gland).
- Anterior pituitary (releases multiple hormones into blood).
- Posterior pituitary (releases oxytocin and vasopressin into blood).

❑❑   **What is an example of a gland that has both exocrine and endocrine functions?**

Pancreas.

❑❑   **What are the three major types of hormones?**

1. Peptide hormone (amino acid chains).
2. Steroid hormone (fat soluble).
3. Amino acid-derived hormones (i.e., epinephrine, norepinephrine, dopamine).

❑❑   **What is the major difference in mode of action between a steroid hormone and a peptide hormone?**

A *steroid* hormone acts *directly on the DNA* of the cell. The fat-soluble hormone passes through the cell membrane for direct interaction with the DNA affecting the SYNTHESIS of proteins.
A *peptide* hormone acts through a "*second messenger*". That is, the peptide hormone attaches to a receptor on the plasma membrane. This attachment sets off a series of reactions that lead to the production of a "second messenger" which typically affects the ACTIVITY of enzymes and other proteins in the cell. The protein hormone does not pass through the cell membrane on its own and *does not* act directly on the DNA.

❑❑   **Which work faster, steroid or peptide hormones?**

Peptide hormones act faster than steroid hormones. The mechanism of action of each explains why this is so. The peptide hormone acts directly on the proteins/enzymes of the cell, whereas the steroid hormone must first affect the DNA, then the proteins/enzymes that the affected DNA produces.

❑❑   **What two hormones (produced into the hypothalamus) are released from the *posterior* pituitary gland?**

1. Oxytocin.
2. Vasopressin (antidiuretic hormone [ADH]).

❑❑   **What are the hormones released from the *anterior* pituitary gland?**

1. Thyroid stimulating hormone (TSH)
2. Adrenocorticotropic hormone (ACTH)
3. Follicle stimulating hormone (FSH)
4. Luteinizing hormone (LH)
5. Growth hormone
6. Prolactin

❏❏ **Name the hormone that:**

1. **Stimulates uterine muscle contraction (childbirth)**
2. **Stimulates ovulation**
3. **Stimulates production of sperm**
4. **Stimulates production of cortisol**
5. **Increases metabolic function**
6. **Stimulates milk production**
7. **Causes reabsorption of water and urea in collecting duct of kidney**
8. **Decreases blood glucose by transporting glucose into cells**
9. **Increases serum calcium levels**
10. **Decreases serum calcium levels**
11. **Suppresses secretion of insulin and glucagon**

1. Oxytocin
2. Luteinizing hormone (LH)
3. Luteinizing hormone (LH)
4. Adrenocorticotropic hormone (ACTH)
5. Thyroid hormone
6. Prolactin
7. Antidiuretic hormone (ADH) or vasopressin
8. Insulin
9. Parathyroid hormone
10. Calcitonin
11. Somatostatin

❏❏ **Where is oxytocin produced? Stored? Secreted? What is the function of oxytocin?**

Oxytocin is produced in the hypothalamus. It is then transported, stored, and secreted from the posterior pituitary gland. Oxytocin stimulates *uterine muscle contraction* and mammary gland cells.

❏❏ **Oxytocin stimulates uterine muscle contraction. In turn, uterine muscle contraction stimulates oxytocin. What type of feedback system is this?**

Positive feedback.

❏❏ **What hormone raises blood calcium levels? What is the mechanism?**

Parathyroid hormone. Parathyroid hormone (released from the parathyroid gland) activates osteoclasts in bone. Osteoclasts (see musculoskeletal section) cause the resorption of bone (breaks down) and calcium is released into the blood.

Also note that parathyroid hormone enhances calcium absorption across intestines and reabsorption of calcium in the kidney.

❏❏ **What hormone increases blood sugar levels? Where is this hormone released from?**

Glucagon. Glucagon is released from the pancreas and stimulates breakdown of glycogen (storage form of sugar) to glucose in the liver. Thus, blood sugar levels increase.

❏❏ **What hormone decreases blood sugar levels? Where is this hormone released from?**

Insulin. Insulin, which is released from the pancreas, causes sugar in the blood to be taken up into cells. It causes an increase in glycogen (storage form) in the liver.

❏❏ **What hormones are released in a "fight or flight" situation? Where are they released from?**

The adrenal medulla releases epinephrine and norepinephrine into the blood. These hormones have a number of effects on target organs serving to prepare the body for fight or flight.

❏❏ **Does the adrenal medulla release predominately epinephrine or norepinephrine?**

Epinephrine (80%).

❏❏ **A patient with a history of asthma presents to the emergency department with wheezing and shortness of breath. The patient receives albuterol (a medicine that stimulates the bronchioles to dilate). The patient also receives steroids that are given to decrease inflammation in the lungs. The patient begins to improve within minutes and thanks the physician for the dose of steroids that he believes saved his life. Is this true?**

No. Remember, steroids are hormones that must first act at the nucleus of the cell by acting on the DNA and affecting the proteins/enzymes that the DNA produces. The albuterol acts immediately to help, but the steroids need several hours to work.

❏❏ **High plasma levels of thyroxine inhibit the pituitary gland from secreting thyroid stimulating hormone (TSH). This decreases the secretion of thyroxine from the thyroid gland. What type of feedback is this?**

Negative feedback.

NERVOUS SYSTEM

❑❑ **Name the two major categories which divide the human nervous system.**

1. *Central* nervous system.
2. *Peripheral* nervous system.

❑❑ **What makes up the central nervous system?**

Brain and spinal cord.

❑❑ **What are the two major divisions of the peripheral nervous system?**

1. *Afferent* division.
2. *Efferent* division.

❑❑ **What is the afferent division of the peripheral nervous system?**

The afferent division is the *sensory* input for the nervous system. The afferent (sensory) division receives input from receptors in the periphery. The impulse travels from the peripheral receptors to the central nervous system.

❑❑ **What is the efferent division of the peripheral nervous system?**

The efferent division is the motor portion of the peripheral nervous system. The efferent (motor) division sends messages from the central nervous system to the periphery.

Memory tip: Efferent = Exit (the spinal cord).

Safety tip: In my experience, many students get confused with introns and extrons (see section on DNA). One reason is that the E for "exit" mnemonic for the efferent nervous system is mixed up with extrons. Extrons do NOT "exit" from RNA, introns do.

❑❑ **What are the two subdivisions of the *efferent* division?**

1. *Autonomic* nervous system.
2. *Somatic* nervous system.

❑❑ **What are the two divisions of the autonomic nervous system?**

1. *Sympathetic* nervous system.
2. *Parasympathetic* nervous system.

❏❏ **What is a neuron? What are the three structural components of a neuron?**

A neuron (or nerve cell) is the functional unit of the nervous system. A neuron is composed of:

1. Dendrite.
2. Cell body.
3. Axon.

❏❏ **Place the following in the correct nervous system (i.e., peripheral or central):**

1. 12 cranial nerves
2. 33 spinal nerves
3. Speech centers
4. Pain receptors

1. Peripheral nervous system (note that CN II is technically considered part of CNS).
2. Peripheral nervous system.
3. Central nervous system (brain).
4. Peripheral nervous system (afferent division).

❏❏ **The cell bodies of the afferent nervous system (sensory) are found where?**

The dorsal root ganglion.

❏❏ **The cell bodies of the efferent nervous system (motor) are found where?**

The ventral horn.

❏❏ **Is the afferent (sensory) nervous system a one-neuron or two-neuron relay system?**

One-neuron—from the periphery to the central nervous system.

❏❏ **Is the efferent (motor) nervous system a one-neuron or two-neuron relay system?**

The efferent nervous system can be *either* a one-neuron or two-neuron relay depending on which section of the efferent division. The somatic division consists of one neuron from the central nervous system to the periphery (skeletal muscle). The autonomic division is a two-neuron system from the central nervous system to ganglia, and then from the ganglia to the target organ.

❑❑ **What is an interneuron?**

Interneurons are located within the central nervous system. They account for 99% of all neurons! The specific roles, connections, and neurotransmitters are thankfully beyond the scope of the MCAT. Just know that they exist and that they allow for communication between neurons WITHIN the CNS.

❑❑ **What is the major differentiating factor between the somatic and the autonomic nervous systems?**

Somatic nervous system: innervates skeletal muscle.
Autonomic nervous system: innervates smooth muscle, cardiac muscle, and glands.

❑❑ **Is the somatic nervous system voluntary or involuntary?**

The somatic nervous system is generally a *voluntarily* controlled system. Of note (but probably not important for the MCAT), exceptions exist such as reflexes. A reflex is not voluntary, yet it is part of the somatic nervous system since skeletal muscle is innervated.

❑❑ **Is the autonomic nervous system voluntary or involuntary?**

The autonomic nervous system is generally an *involuntary* system. Exceptions do occur, such as Buddhist monks (among others) who can intentionally control heart rate and such. Again, the definition of autonomic depends on the target organ or muscle that is innervated, namely, smooth muscle, cardiac muscle, or glands.

❑❑ **What are the two parts of the autonomic nervous system?**

Sympathetic nervous system and parasympathetic nervous system.

❑❑ **How can the functions of the sympathetic and parasympathic nervous systems generally be differentiated?**

The sympathetic nervous system is involved in "fight or flight" functions, whereas the parasympathetic nervous system is involved in "rest and relaxation" or "rest and digest" functions.

❑❑ **Label the following with sympathetic, parasympathetic, both, or neither:**

1. **Fight or flight.**
2. **Two-neuron relay.**
3. **Relay in sympathetic chain.**
4. **Relay close to or on target organ.**
5. **Maintain homeostasis.**
6. **Arises from thoraco-lumbar levels of spinal cord.**
7. **Arises from cranial-sacral levels of spinal cord.**

1. Sympathetic.
2. Both.
3. Sympathetic.
4. Parasympathetic.
5. Both.
6. Sympathetic.
7. Parasympathetic.

❑❑ What is the difference between a ganglion and a nucleus?

A nucleus is a bundle of cell bodies in the central nervous system. A ganglion is a bundle of cell bodies located in the periphery. Ganglia receive neurons from the central nervous system (pre-ganglionic neurons). These neurons release their neurotransmitters into the synaptic cleft and stimulate the second neuron (post-ganglionic neurons). The cell bodies of the post-ganglionic neurons are located in the ganglia. The post-ganglionic neurons then go to the target organ.

❑❑ Where are the sympathetic ganglia located?

The sympathetic ganglia are located very close to the spinal cord in the sympathetic chain. Here they synapse with each other and send signals to the target organs. Thus, they have a short pre-ganglionic segment and a long post-ganglionic segment.

❑❑ Where are the parasympathetic ganglia located?

Parasympathetic ganglia are located on or very near their target organ. Thus, they have long pre-ganglionic segments and short post-ganglionic segments.

❑❑ Which system (sympathetic or parasympathetic) offers more diverse function? Why?

The sympathetic system allows for more diverse function. This is accomplished via the many communications in the sympathetic ganglion. The parasympathetic system does not communicate in this manner.

❑❑ How does the nervous system transmit signals?

The nervous system transmits signals by:
1. Action potentials (along the axon).
2. Neurotransmitters (at the synaptic cleft).

❑❑ What is a neurotransmitter?

A neurotransmitter is typically an amino acid derivative (i.e., norepinephrine, epinephrine, acetylcholine) which is released from the synaptic knob of a neuron. The neurotransmitter traverses the synaptic cleft and either excites or inhibits the adjoining neuron or target organ/muscle.

❑❑ **What ion is released into the synaptic knob in order to stimulate the release of neurotransmitter into the synaptic cleft?**

Calcium. The influx of calcium into the synaptic knob causes vesicles (structures which contain neurotransmitter) to extrude neurotransmitter into the synaptic cleft via exocytosis.

❑❑ **What are the neurotransmitter (s) used in the parasympathetic system?**

Acetylcholine is used in *both* synapses of the parasympathetic system.

❑❑ **What is the neurotransmitter (s) used in the sympathetic system?**

Acetylcholine is released from pre- to post-ganglionic neurons.
Norepinephrine is released from the post-ganglionic neurons to the target organ.

❑❑ **At rest, is the inside of a neuron more or less negative than the outside?**

More negative.

❑❑ **At rest, is the [K⁺] higher on the inside or the outside of the neuron?**

Inside.

❑❑ **At rest, is the [Na⁺] higher on the inside or the outside of the neuron?**

Outside.

❑❑ **How is the concentration gradient of potassium and sodium maintained in the neuron?**

By a selectively permeable membrane and through use of the sodium-potassium pump.

❑❑ **What is the refractory period?**

The time immediately after an action potential when it is impossible to initiate another action potential.

❑❑ **What are two structural aspects of a neuron which affect conduction speed?**

1. Diameter of the neuron.
2. Myelination.

❑❑ **How does diameter affect the speed of conduction?**

The *larger* the diameter, the *faster* the speed.

❏❏   **What is myelination?**

Myelination is the covering around a neuron much like insulation on a wire. Like the insulation on a metal wire, no electric current is conducted. Thus, electric current is conducted by skipping over the insulated or myelinated portions to "nodes" where there is no myelin. These nodes are termed "nodes of Ranvier."

❏❏   **What type of supporting cell forms the myelin sheath in the peripheral nervous system?**

Schwann cell.

❏❏   **What type of supporting cell forms the myelin sheath in the central nervous system?**

Oligodendroctyes.

❏❏   **What is saltatory conduction?**

This is the term used to describe nerve conduction that takes place via the nodes of Ranvier. The nerve transmission jumps from node to node. Since the myelinated (insulated) segments are "skipped," this significantly speeds nerve conduction. Interestingly, "saltatory" is derived from the Latin word "saltare" which means "to jump".

❏❏   **How are olfaction (i.e., smell) and taste sensed by the nervous system?**

Both the olfactory and taste systems use receptors to bind to molecules. The molecules are either gases (for olfaction) or in solution (for taste).

❏❏   **Trace the path of sound through the ear, from the outer ear to the brain.**

Sound (in the form of moving air molecules) enters the outer ear, travels through the auditory canal, and impacts on the tympanic membrane (i.e., the ear drum). This causes the membrane to vibrate, and these vibrations are amplified as they travel through the ossicles (i.e., the tiny bones of the middle ear). These amplified vibrations cause the oval window to vibrate and this is translated to movement of the fluid (called the endolymph) inside the cochlea. The movement of endolymph stimulates hair cells which can depolarize and transmit an electrical nerve impulse to the brain.

❏❏   **Trace the path of light through the eye to the brain.**

Photons of light that enter the eye pass through the cornea, the anterior chamber, the pupil, the lens, and the posterior chamber, and impact on the retina. The impacting photons stimulate the photoreceptors (i.e., the rods and cones) on the retina. These cells then transmit electrical nerve impulses to the brain.

CELL DIVISION

❑❑ **What does the quote "Omnis cellula e cellula" mean?**

"All cells from cells." This is a summary statement that Rudolf Virchow made when he put forth the cell theory in 1855.

❑❑ **What are the two major stages of the cell cycle?**

Interphase and M phase (mitosis and cytokinesis).

❑❑ **What takes place during interphase?**

This is the phase in which much *cellular activity* takes place. Most of the cell cycle (90%) is spent in interphase. During interphase the chromosomes and DNA divide.

❑❑ **What are the three phases of interphase?**

G_1, S phase, G_2.

❑❑ **During which phase of interphase does the DNA divide?**

S phase.

❑❑ **A cell is suddenly halted just prior to entering mitosis. What phase of the cell cycle did this cell enter?**

G_0 phase.

❑❑ **What are the phases of mitosis?**

Four phases:
1. Prophase.
2. Metaphase.
3. Anaphase.
4. Telophase.

❑❑ **A scientist poisons a cell when all of the chromosomes are lined up in the midline of the mitotic spindle.   What phase of the mitosis is this?**

Metaphase.

❑❑ **In what phase of mitosis do chromosomes condense and spindles form?**

Prophase.

❑❑ **What type of structure is the mitotic spindle made of?**

The mitotic spindle is made from *microtubules*.

❑❑ **After telophase is complete, what other process must occur to finish the division of the cell?**

The previously named steps represent division of the chromosomes and equal disbursement of the chromatids. BUT, the cell still needs to be completely divided. That is, the *cytoplasm* must divide. This takes place following telophase by a process termed *cytokinesis*.

❑❑ **Match the mitotic structure with the appropriate description:**

a) **Small cylindrical bodies located just outside the nucleus which duplicate and migrate to opposite poles.**
b) **Two of these are called twins, and together they make up a chromosome.**
c) **A cytoskeletal structure that forms the scaffolding for chromosome separation.**
d) **A system of microtubules that surround and radiate out from the centrioles.**
e) **Associated chromatids are connected to each other by these.**
f) **These are found at the ends of each chromosome.**
g) **These connect the centromeres to the poles.**

1. **Kinetochores**
2. **Centromeres**
3. **Chromatids**
4. **Spindles**
5. **Asters**
6. **Telomeres**
7. **Centrioles**

1. g; 2. e; 3. b; 4. c; 5. d; 6. f; 7. a.

❑❑ **How do bacterial cells divide?**

Binary fission. A cell replicates its one and only chromosome. Next, the two chromosomes attach to the plasma wall. The cell elongates and divides, creating two identical cells. This allows for rapid growth (i.e., cells divide exponentially).

❑❑ **Do human cells divide via mitosis or meiosis?**

This is a trick question, as our cells undergo *both* mitosis and meiosis, depending on the type and function of the cell. For example, spermatogonia divide by mitosis prior to beginning their meiotic division to create spermatozoa.

❏❏ **How many chromosomes do bacteria have?**

One.

❏❏ **How many chromosomes does a human cell have?**

All human cells (except sperm and eggs) have 46 chromosomes (23 pairs).

❏❏ **How is bacterial DNA arranged in the cell?**

Bacteria have circular DNA.

REPRODUCTIVE SYSTEM AND DEVELOPMENT

❑❑ **Where does spermatogenesis take place?**

The testes, specifically in the seminiferous tubules.

❑❑ **Trace the path of a spermatozoon after ejaculation from the male (in the vagina) until its union with an ovum.**

Vagina → Uterine cervix (through the cervical opening) → Body of the uterus → Fallopian tube (It is here in the Fallopian tube that the sperm joins with the ovum.)

❑❑ **How do the products of meiosis and mitosis differ?**

Mitosis produces two identical daughter cells from one parent cell. Meiosis produces four haploid daughter cells, each different from the other.

❑❑ **List the stages of spermatogenesis of a single spermatogonium.**

Spermatogonium (2N) → Primary spermatocyte (2N) → 2 Secondary spermatocytes (N) → 4 Spermatids (N) → 4 Spermatozoa (N)

❑❑ **At what stage of meiosis is oogenesis halted until puberty?**

Prophase of meiosis I.

❑❑ **What are the products of oogenesis?**

A mature ovum and up to 3 polar bodies.

❑❑ **What 2 hormones are essential to both spermatogenesis and oogenesis?**

Luteinizing hormone (LH) and follicle-stimulating hormone (FSH).

❑❑ **What structure serves as the site of exchange between the fetus and the mother?**

The placenta.

❑❑   **Into what organ does the placenta implant?**

The uterus.

❑❑   **Match the terms with each description (use each term only once).**

a) **Fertilization**
b) **Gastrulation**
c) **Neurulation**
d) **Blastulation**
e) **Cleavage**

1. **During this stage, the embryo forms the ectoderm and the inner layer.**
2. **During this stage, the embryo forms a fluid-filled cavity called a blastocoele.**
3. **This is the joining of a spermatozoon and an ovum.**
4. **During this stage, the cells of the embryo divide rapidly as it travels down the Fallopian tube.**
5. **During this stage, the notochord is formed.**

1.b; 2.d; 3.a; 4.e; 5.c

❑❑   **Place the stages (a through e) in the above question in order of occurrence.**

Fertilization → Cleavage → Blastulation → Gastrulation → Neurulation.

❑❑   **What are the three primary germ layers of embryonic development?**

Endoderm, mesoderm, and ectoderm.

❑❑   **List some major structures that arise from each primary germ layer.**

See chart below:

Endoderm	Mesoderm	Ectoderm
Thyroid	Bone	Hair
Bladder	Muscle	Nails
Liver	Blood cells	Epidermis
Pancreas	Kidneys	Lens of the eye
Lungs	Gonads	Nervous system
Lining of some internal organs		Epithelium of the nose, mouth, and anus

❏❏ **What is "induction" of developing cells?**

Induction is the process by which cells influence the development of neighboring cells.

❏❏ **What is meant by the "differentiation" of developing cells?**

Differentiation is the process by which cells develop into highly specialized cells and tissues.

GENETICS AND EVOLUTION

❑❑ **What is an allele?**

Alleles are different forms of a given gene. For example, a gene for eye color may have one allele coding for blue eyes and one allele coding for brown eyes.

❑❑ **T/F: When pairs of alleles separate, they do so in a random fashion.**

True. This is Mendel's first law.

❑❑ **Assume that a flower has a gene for the color of its petals. The dominant allele is for red petals (P) and the recessive allele is for white petals (p). If two parents are crossed that are both Pp, then what fraction of offspring will be PP? Pp? pp? What fraction will be red?**

Set up a Punnett square.

	P	P
P	PP	Pp
p	Pp	pp

The fraction of offspring with PP = ¼; Pp = ½; pp = ¼.
The fraction of offspring that are red is ¾. (Only pp genotype offspring will be white.)

❑❑ **What is the Hardy-Weinberg law?**

Under certain ideal conditions, the frequency of each allele in a population remains unchanged. (These conditions are never perfectly met in the real world.)

❑❑ **What is the Hardy-Weinberg equilibrium?**

$p^2 + 2pq + q^2 = 1$ where p = one allele and q = another allele.

p^2 = frequency of dominant homozygotes
$2pq$ = frequency of heterozygotes
q^2 = frequency of recessive homozygotes

❑❑ **What are the sex chromosomes in a normal human male? In a female?**

Male = XY, Female = XX

❑❑ **On which chromosome are sex-linked genes found?**

On the X chromosome.

❑❑ **Define fitness with respect to natural selection.**

Fitness is the ability to succeed in a given environment.

❑❑ **What is meant by the term differential reproduction?**

This means that individuals that are better adapted to their environment will have a greater number of viable offspring than individuals that are less well adapted.

❑❑ **What is the term used to denote the development of a new species?**

Speciation.

RANDOM QUESTIONS

❏❏ **Match the organ with the correct description (answers may be used more than once):**

a) **Gallbladder**
b) **Heart**
c) **Kidney**
d) **Liver**
e) **Lungs**
f) **Pancreas**
g) **Skin**
h) **Stomach**

1. **Regulates blood pressure**
2. **Provides protection, maintains homeostatic functions, helps regulate temperature**
3. **Produces amylase, lipase, and carboxypeptidase**
4. **Produces bile**
5. **Maintains pH of 2-3**
6. **Helps maintains acid-base balance, removes nitrogenous wastes**
7. **Stores bile**

1.c; 2.g; 3.f; 4.d; 5.h; 6.c; 7.a

❏❏ **Why does an alcohol generally require an acid catalyst in order to undergo nucleophilic substitution?**

The acid protonates the ⁻OH and thus forms water. Remember ⁻OH is a BAD leaving group, but H_2O is a GOOD leaving group.

❏❏ **What is the shape of streptococcus pneumonia?**

SPHERICAL. Don't get fooled by the name of an organism. Of course you are NOT expected to know individual types of bacteria. But, you should recognize COCCUS from streptoCOCCUS and recall that COCCUS=SPHERICAL.

❏❏ **What is the shape of bacillus aureus?**

ROD-SHAPED. Again, recognize BACILLUS from this name. BACILLI=ROD-SHAPED.

❑❑ **Where does protein digestion begin?**

Stomach.

❑❑ **If you walk outside on an very hot summer day, what physiologic responses occur in order for you to attempt to stay cool?**

1. Vasodilation: Peripheral blood vessels dilate. This delivers increased supply of blood to periphery. The increased blood supply dissipates heat to the environment.
2. Sweating: Evaporation of sweat reduces body heat.
3. Panting: Supposedly increased respiratory rate will help give off heat. This occurs in certain animal species but whether this occurs in humans is more controversial.

❑❑ **If you walk outside on a cold day, what physiologic response occurs in order to help conserve heat?**

1. Vasoconstriction: Peripheral blood vessels (arterioles) constrict and thereby decrease blood supply to the periphery. The decreased blood volume results in decreased heat dissipated to the environment. In addition, blood is shunted to the important central organs, namely, the brain and the heart.
2. Shivering: This act increases metabolism and thus causes increased production of heat.

❑❑ **Which part of the digestive tract accounts for most of digestion?**

The small intestine has the LARGEST SURFACE AREA of all digestive organs and is involved in digestion of carbohydrates, fats, and proteins. Thus, this organ accounts for most of digestion.

❑❑ **What is the major difference between facilitated transport and active transport?**

Active transport REQUIRES ENERGY whereas facilitated transport (a type of passive transport) does not. Both types of transport involve carrier proteins and therefore both have a saturation point (all carriers are being used and thus a maximum velocity is reached).

❑❑ **After running a marathon, what major biochemical product do you expect to accumulate in the muscles?**

Lactic acid.

❑❑ **Hyperventilation causes a decrease in...?**

Carbon dioxide. An increase in gas exchange in the lungs causes more carbon dioxide to be expelled.

❏❏ **As a patient slips into hypovolemic shock (low blood volume), what will happen to his/her heart rate?**

INCREASES. Remember that a significant decrease in blood volume causes a reflexive increase in the heart rate in order to compensate for the decreased blood supply to the tissues.

❏❏ **When an action potential arrives at a synaptic knob, an ion gate opens and an ion rushes in. What is the ion?**

CALCIUM. Remember, an action potential stimulates calcium channels to open and calcium rushes into the synaptic knob. The calcium then causes the vesicles to release their contents into the synaptic cleft by way of exocytosis.

❏❏ **What is contained inside the vesicles mentioned above?**

NEUROTRANSMITTERS. A neurotransmitter is a substance which serves as a chemical messenger for the nervous system. They are exuded into a synaptic cleft via exocytosis. Next they bind to the membrane on the other side of the synaptic cleft called the postsynaptic membrane. The postsynaptic membrane may be another neuron or a muscle.

❏❏ **Ovulation is stimulated by what hormone?**

Luteinizing hormone (LH).

❏❏ **What is the function of epithelial cells?**

Epithelial cells line the skin and internal organs and provide protection from microbes, mechanical insults, etc.

❏❏ **What is the difference between simple and stratified epithelium?**

Simple epithelium is one cell layer thick, while stratified epithelium is many cell layers thick.

GENERAL CHEMISTRY

THE BASICS

❑❑ **What is an atom?**

This is the smallest component of an element that has all of the chemical properties of that element.

❑❑ **What is an element?**

An element is formed from many atoms of only one type and cannot be broken down by chemical or physical means. The atoms of an element show similar chemical properties.

❑❑ **What are the three types of sub-atomic particles?**

Protons, electrons, and neutrons.

❑❑ **What is a proton?**

A *positively* charged particle in the nucleus of an element.

❑❑ **What is an electron?**

A *negatively* charged particle located in a "cloud-like" arrangement outside the nucleus of an element.

❑❑ **T/F: A hydrogen ion (H^+) is a single proton.**

True. Hydrogen contains one proton and one electron. Taking away an electron creates H^+ that contains only a single proton.

❑❑ **What is a neutron?**

A particle with *no charge* located in the nucleus of an element.

❑❑ **What is the nucleus of an atom composed of?**

The nucleus is composed of neutrons and protons.

❑❑ **How many electrons are in Na? Protons? Refer to a periodic table.**

11, 11.

❑❑ **How many electrons are in Na^+? Protons?**

10, 11.

❑❑ **T/F: The mass of a proton is virtually equal to the mass of a neutron.**

True.

❑❑ **T/F: The mass of an electron is virtually equal to the mass of a proton.**

False. An electron has a much smaller mass (1/1800) than that of a proton or a neutron.

❑❑ **T/F: The charge of an electron is equal (and opposite) to the charge of a proton.**

True.

❑❑ **Which of the following are located in the nucleus of the atom: protons, neutrons, or electrons?**

Protons and neutrons are located within the nucleus. Electrons are found in shells surrounding the nucleus.

❑❑ **How is the periodic table organized?**

The periodic table is organized by the *atomic numbers* of the elements.

❑❑ **What is the atomic number?**

The atomic number is the number of protons in the nucleus of an atom.

❑❑ **What is the mass number?**

The mass number is determined by the total mass of the protons and neutrons in the nucleus.

❑❑ **What is the difference between atomic weight and molecular weight?**

Atomic weight refers to the average mass of a mole of an element in the periodic table. The atomic weights of each element are listed in the periodic table. *Molecular weight* refers to the weight of a *compound*. This is determined by adding the atomic weights of each of the elements in the compound.

❑❑ **Calculate the molecular weight of the following:**

$$C_2H_6.$$

First, look up the atomic weights of both carbon and hydrogen (carbon = 12, hydrogen = 1). Then, multiply the atomic weight of each by the subscript. Thus,

Molecular Weight = (12 x 2) + (1 x 6) = 30

❑❑ **What is the difference between atomic weight and atomic number?**

The *atomic weight* is the weight of one mole of an element in the periodic table. The *atomic number* of an element represents the number of protons that the element contains. Thus, the atomic weight and atomic number are usually related, as most of the weight of an element is derived from the weight of protons...BUT this is only a broad generalization. ISOTOPES illustrate this difference (see next question).

❑❑ **What are isotopes?**

Isotopes are two molecules which have the *same atomic number* (number of protons) but *different atomic weight* (different number of neutrons which alter weight).

❑❑ **Terms for the horizontal line of elements on the periodic table:**

Row or period.

❑❑ **Term for the vertical line of elements on the periodic table:**

Column.

❑❑ **In general, going left to right along a row on the periodic table, what happens to:**
   Electronegativity
   Electron affinity
   Ion dissociation energy
   Atomic radius

From left to right (across a row):
   Electronegativity: INCREASES
   Electron affinity: INCREASES
   Ion dissociation energy: INCREASES
   Atomic radius: DECREASES

❑❑ **In general, going down a column on the periodic table, what happens to:**
   Electronegativity
   Electron affinity
   Ionic dissociation energy
   Atomic radius

From top to bottom (down a column):
   Electronegativity: DECREASES
   Electron affinity: DECREASES
   Ion dissociation energy: DECREASES
   Atomic radius: INCREASES

❑❑ **What is electronegativity?**

Electronegativity is a measure of the tendency of an atom to draw electrons to itself in a chemical bond.

❑❑ **What is electron affinity?**

Electron affinity is a measure of the amount of energy associated with a gaseous atom or group of atoms gaining an electron.

❑❑ **What is ionization energy?**

This is the amount of energy required to remove an electron from the outer shell of an element and thus create an ion.

❑❑ **Why does ionization energy increase going from left to right on the periodic table?**

Going from left to right on the periodic table, the positive charge of the nucleus increases and the atomic radius decreases. The increasing positive charge increases the energy needed to remove a negatively charged electron from the outer shell.

❑❑ **Why does ionization energy decrease going down a column in the periodic table?**

Going down a column in the periodic table, an additional shell of electrons is added. Each element in the column contains the same number of electrons in the outer shell. Thus, the addition of an entire shell of the same number of electrons decreases the attraction of the outer shell electron to the proton in the nucleus. Ionization energy (i.e., energy needed to remove the electron) is therefore decreased.

❑❑ **When is radiation emitted from electrons?**

When an electron moves to an orbit of lower energy from an orbit of higher energy, radiation (energy) is emitted in the form of a photon.

❏❏ **What is the difference between empirical and molecular formulas?**

An empirical formula is the chemical formula of a compound expressed as the smallest ratio of whole numbers (e.g., CH). The molecular formula is the actual chemical composition (e.g., C_6H_6) of the compound.

❏❏ **A compound contains 12.0 grams of carbon, 2.0 grams of hydrogen, and 48.0 grams of oxygen. What is the empirical formula for this compound?**

Use the periodic table to find that hydrogen = 1 gram/mole, carbon = 12 grams/mole, and oxygen = 16 grams/mole. Thus,

Hydrogen = 2 grams / 1 gram/mole = 2 moles.

Carbon = 12 grams / 12 grams/mole = 1 mole.

Oxygen = 48 grams / 16 grams/mole = 3 moles.

The complete molecule therefore equals = H_2CO_3.

❏❏ **How many miles are in 20 kilometers? Wait! Do I have to know this?**

No! Don't waste time learning/memorizing conversions from the metric to the American system. All questions will be in metric units. Of course you *do* need to know how to convert between different units within the metric system.

❏❏ **Calculate the following conversions:**
A) 200 kilograms = ? grams
B) 10 grams = ? kilograms
C) 10 liters = ? milliliters
D) 100 centimeters = ? kilometers

A) 200,000 grams; B) 0.01 kilograms; C) 10,000 milliliters; D) 0.001 kilometers.

❏❏ **What is a mole?**

A mole is defined by 6.02×10^{23} atoms. This number is based on the number of atoms in 12 grams of carbon. By using a mole to define 6.02×10^{23} atoms, very large numbers can be easily managed.

❏❏ **Calculate the number of moles in 34 grams of NH_3.**

The number of moles is calculated as follows:

Nitrogen   =   14 grams/mole
Hydrogen   =   1 gram/mole x 3
Total   =   17 grams/mole

$\dfrac{34 \text{ grams } NH_3}{\dfrac{\text{mole}}{17 \text{ grams}}}$ ÷ $\dfrac{34 \text{ grams } NH_3}{\text{mole}}$ x $\dfrac{? \text{ moles } NH_3}{17 \text{ grams}}$ = 2 moles of NH_3

? moles NH_3

❏❏ **Calculate the number of grams of carbon in 3 moles of methane (CH_4).**

Carbon = 12 grams/mole

$\dfrac{12 \text{ grams of carbon}}{\text{mole}}$ X   3 moles = 36 grams of carbon

❏❏ **What is the percent, by mass, of carbon in CO_2?**

Percent mass of an individual component of a compound can be determined by dividing the molecular weight of that compound by the total molecular weight. Thus,

$\dfrac{\text{Molecular weight of carbon}}{\text{Molecular weight of } CO_2}$ = $\dfrac{12 \text{ grams/mole}}{44 \text{ grams/mole}}$ = .27 = 27%

BONDING

❏❏ **What is the difference between a compound and a mixture?**

A compound can be broken down by chemical means, and a mixture can be broken down by physical means.

❏❏ **What is the difference between an ionic and a covalent bond?**

An ionic bond is formed from the charges created after a *transfer* of electrons from one element to another. For example, sodium transfers an electron to chloride. This electron creates a negative charge on the chloride. The loss of the electron leaves a positive charge on the sodium. The negative and positive charges attract, thus forming an ionic bond.

A covalent bond is formed through the *sharing* of electrons between two elements. For example, HCl forms a covalent bond. Hydrogen has one electron in its outer shell (needs two to fill the shell), whereas chloride has seven (needs eight to fill the shell). Hydrogen shares its electron with chloride, and chloride shares one of its electrons with hydrogen. Through this sharing, both maintain full outer shells of electrons.

❏❏ **Between what two types of elements do ionic bonds form? Covalent bonds?**

Ionic bonds form between a *metal and a non-metal*, whereas *covalent* bonds form between *two non-metals*.

❏❏ **What is partial ionic character?**

This is the "gray area" of bonding. In the real world of molecules, bonds are not fully ionic or fully covalent, but represent a mix of the two. Those that tend to be mostly ionic are described as such, and vice versa for covalent.

❏❏ **What is a hydrogen bond?**

A hydrogen bond is an intermolecular bond formed between a hydrogen atom of one substance and an atom of another element which carries a partial negative charge. For example:

$$CH_3\text{-}CH_2\text{-}CH_2\text{-}O \text{———} H \quad NH_2 \text{———} CH_3$$

In this example, the partial positive charge of the hydrogen is attracted to the partial negative charge of the NH_2.

❑❑ **What are the three possible elements that can form hydrogen bonds?**

The three elements are Fluorine, Oxygen, and Nitrogen.
Memory tip: Think of a "FON bond".

❑❑ **What are the intermolecular forces formed by weak interactions between molecules?**

Van der Waals forces.

❑❑ **Rank the following bonds in order from strongest to weakest: covalent, ionic, hydrogen bonding, van der Waals forces.**

Covalent > ionic > hydrogen > van der Waals.

❑❑ **Is energy needed to break or to form bonds?**

Energy is needed to *break* bonds, whereas *energy* is *given off* when bonds are *formed*. This simple statement is often confused. Thus, take a moment to understand as well as memorize this.

❑❑ **Which is the strongest kind of bonding?**

COVALENT bonding.

❑❑ **What is bond dissociation energy?**

Bond dissociation energy is the average amount of energy per mole needed to break a bond.

❑❑ **List the following in order of the length of bonds from longest to shortest:**

$$F_2, Cl_2, Br_2, I_2$$

I_2 (longest) → Br_2 → Cl_2 → F_2

❑❑ **Can any comparison be made between the length of a C-H bond in ethane and a C-H bond in adenine?**

Yes, a specific type of bond varies only slightly in length/bond energy when in different molecules. Thus, generalizations/estimations of bond length and energy may be made about a multitude of different molecules.

❑❑ **When a bond is formed, does it require energy or give off energy?**

Bond formation *gives off* energy.

EQUILIBRIUM

□□ **What does it mean to be "at equilibrium?"**

At equilibrium, the rate of the forward reaction and the rate of the backward reaction are equivalent. The equilibrium constant, K, is the ratio of products to reactants when the forward and backward reaction rates are equivalent.

K (equilibrium constant) = products/reactants.

□□ **T/F: At equilibrium, the chemical reaction is finally at rest.**

False. As noted above, at equilibrium, the forward and the backward reaction rates are equivalent. This does not mean they are at rest. To the contrary, the reaction is undergoing constant movement from reactant to product and vice versa. Thus, the term "dynamic" is often used to describe equilibrium.

□□ **What is the equilibrium constant (K) for the following reaction?**

$$2 \text{ HCl (g)} + \text{H}_2\text{O (aq)} \longleftrightarrow \text{H}_3\text{O}^+ \text{(aq)} + \text{Cl}_2 \text{(g)}$$

The equilibrium constant (K) is the ratio of the products to the reactants. The number of moles (coefficient) of a molecule becomes an exponent (superscript) in the equation such that 2 HCl becomes $[\text{HCl}]^2$. Thus,

$$K_{(eq)} = [\text{H}_3\text{O}^+] [\text{Cl}_2] / [\text{HCl}]^2 [\text{H}_2\text{O}]$$

□□ **What is the equilibrium constant (K) for the following reaction?**

$$\text{O}_2\text{(g)} + 2\text{H}_2\text{O(l)} \longleftrightarrow 2\text{H}_2\text{O}_2\text{(aq)}$$

This question tests the concept that liquids and solids are not placed into the equilibrium equation. Only aqueous solutions and gases make up the equilibrium equation. Thus, the equilibrium equation for this question would be:

$$K = \frac{[\text{H}_2\text{O}_2]^2}{\text{P}_{\text{O}2}}$$

❏❏ **For the following values of K, determine whether the reactants or the products would be greater:**

1) K = 1.5   2) K = 1.0   3) K = .5

1) Products are greater; 2) Products/reactants equivalent; 3) Reactants are greater.

❏❏ **Is equilibrium (K) a state property?**

Yes. K is determined by the final outcome of the ratio of products to reactants and not by the steps needed to get to that point.

❏❏ **When K(eq) = 1, what is the G for the reaction?**

When K (eq) = 1, the G of the reaction = 0 (see thermodynamics section).

❏❏ **What is Le Chatelier's principle?**

Le Chatelier's principle states that if a stress is applied to a system at equilibrium, the system will shift in the direction that minimizes the effects of that stress.

❏❏ **Which way will the following reaction proceed if more of compound A is added?**

$$A + B \leftrightarrow C + D$$

If more A is added, the reaction will shift to the right. Remember, adding a substance shifts the reaction *away* from the side of addition.

❏❏ **Which way will the following reaction proceed if compound B is removed?**

$$A + B \leftrightarrow C + D$$

If compound B is removed, the reaction will shift to the left. Remember, removing a substance shifts the reaction *toward* the side of removal.

❏❏ **In which direction will an endothermic reaction proceed if heat is added?**

If heat is added to an endothermic reaction, the reaction will proceed to the right. A good way to envision this is to actually add heat to the reaction equation such as:

$$Heat + A + B \leftrightarrow C + D$$

An endothermic reaction requires heat, and thus heat is added to the left side of the equation. An exothermic reaction gives off heat, and thus heat is added to the right side of the equation. *Increase* in heat shifts the reaction *away from the side that contains heat* in the equation.

❑❑ **In which direction will the following reaction proceed if the pressure of the system is increased?**

$$2\ NO(g)\ +\ O_2(g)\ \leftrightarrow\ 2\ NO_2(g)$$

The reaction will shift to the right. An increase in pressure shifts the reaction *toward* the side with the *fewer total moles of gas.*

❑❑ **Which way will an exothermic reaction proceed if heat is added?**

If heat is added to an exothermic reaction, then the reaction will proceed to the left. As indicated in a previous question, adding heat to the appropriate side of the reaction may help to envision this.

$$A\ +\ B\ \leftrightarrow\ C\ +\ D\ +\ Heat$$

❑❑ **The following reaction represents the carbon dioxide-bicarbonate buffer system in the human body. How will hyperventilation affect the reaction?**

$$CO_2\ +\ H_2O\ \leftrightarrow\ H_2CO_3\ \leftrightarrow\ HCO_3^-\ +\ H^+$$

Hyperventilation causes CO_2 to decrease. Thus, the reaction would shift to the left.

❑❑ **What is the reaction quotient (Q)?**

The reaction quotient is the ratio of products to reactants at a particular time, not necessarily equilibrium.

❑❑ **When Q is greater than K, which way does the reaction proceed in order to reach equilibrium?**

When Q is greater than K, this means the ratio of products to reactants is greater at that moment (Q) than at equilibrium (K). Thus, the reaction will proceed to the left (decrease product/increase reactants) in order to reach equilibrium.

❑❑ **When K is greater than Q, which way does the reaction proceed in order to reach equilibrium?**

When K is greater than Q, this means the ratio of products to reactants is greater at equilibrium (K) than at this moment (Q). Thus, the reaction proceeds from left to right (decrease reactants/increase products) in order to reach equilibrium.

❑❑ **What is the equilibrium equation for the following reaction?**

$$PCl_5(g)\ \leftrightarrow\ PCl_3(g)\ +\ Cl_2(g)$$

$K = [PCl_3][Cl_2]/[PCl_5]$

❏❏   **How (i.e., what formula) is the equilibrium constant related to Gibbs free energy (G)?**

$\Delta G = ^-RT\ln K$

❏❏   **If K = 1, what does ΔG equal?**

When K = 1, $\Delta G = 0$

❏❏   **When K < 1, what is ΔG?   What about K > 1?**

When K < 1, $\Delta G > 0$
When K > 1, $\Delta G < 0$

THERMODYNAMICS

❑❑ **What is heat capacity?**

Heat capacity is the amount of heat required to raise the temperature of a substance by one degree Kelvin or Celsius.

❑❑ **What is molar heat capacity?**

Molar heat capacity is the amount of heat required to raise the temperature of one mole of a substance by one degree Kelvin or Celsius.

❑❑ **What is specific heat capacity?**

Specific heat capacity is the amount of heat required to raise the temperature of one gram of a substance by one degree Kelvin or Celsius.

❑❑ **What is the formula for determining specific heat capacity?**

$q = n\, c_p\, \Delta t$ where q = heat absorbed, n = moles of substance, c_p = heat capacity (at constant pressure), and t = temperature.

❑❑ **What is a state function?**

A state function is one that is independent of pathway. Thus, a state function depends only on the current system (i.e., state) and not the history/pathway that was required to get to that point.

❑❑ **Name some examples of state functions.**

Examples of state functions include pressure, volume, temperature, enthalpy, entropy, internal energy, and free energy.

❑❑ **Name examples of nonstate functions.**

Examples of nonstate functions include work and heat. Imagine the work required to carry a suitcase up a staircase. In the process, imagine the suitcase falling back down the staircase, requiring additional work to get to the top. Thus, work is dependent on the pathway and not just the state.

❑❑ **What is the first law of thermodynamics?**

The first law of thermodynamics, sometimes called the law of conservation of energy, states that in any process, energy is neither created nor destroyed.

❑❑ **What is enthalpy?**

Enthalpy is the heat content of a substance. At a constant pressure, the heat absorbed by a system is equal to the change in enthalpy. This change in heat energy is symbolized as ΔH.

❑❑ **What is the difference between an endothermic and an exothermic reaction?**

An exothermic reaction releases heat energy into the environment. An endothermic reaction needs heat energy to be put into the reaction.
- *Exo*thermic: *Gives off* energy.
- *Endo*thermic: Energy is *put into* the reaction.

❑❑ **What will the sign (positive or negative) of enthalpy be for an exothermic reaction? For an endothermic reaction?**

As noted, enthalpy is symbolized by ΔH and represents the change in heat energy that takes place during a reaction. An *endothermic* reaction means that heat energy is *put into* the reaction (ΔH is *POSITIVE*). An *exothermic* reaction means that heat energy is *given off* in a reaction (ΔH is *NEGATIVE*).
ENDOTHERMIC: +
EXOTHERMIC: -

❑❑ **Is the following an endothermic or an exothermic reaction?**

$$A + B \rightarrow C + D + heat.$$

This reaction is exothermic because heat is *given off*.

❑❑ **A test tube is cold after the completion of a reaction. Was this an exothermic or endothermic reaction?**

Endothermic. The test tube is cold; therefore the reaction used up heat – hence, endothermic.

❑❑ **Is the following reaction endothermic or exothermic?**

$$NaCl(s) \rightarrow Na^+(aq) + Cl^-(aq) \; \Delta H = {}^+3.9 \; kj$$

Endothermic (Change in enthalpy is positive).

❑❑ **Based on the enthalpy given in the previous question, answer the following:**

$$Na^+(aq) + Cl^-(aq) \rightarrow NaCl(s) \qquad \Delta H = ?$$

⁻3.9 kj. If a reaction is reversed, simply change the sign (+/-) to derive the enthalpy.

❑❑ **What does ΔH^o refer to?**

ΔH^o refers to the change in enthalpy (heat energy) at standard state (25° C or 298.15^o K and 1 atmosphere of pressure).

❑❑ **What does ΔH^o_f refer to?**

ΔH^o_f is the enthalpy of formation. This is the amount of energy (heat) which is given off when a particular compound is formed. For example (see below), to form HCl an enthalpy change of ⁻92.3 occurs.

$$H_2 + Cl_2 \rightarrow HCl \qquad \Delta H^o_f = {}^-92.3$$

❑❑ **What is the heat of formation of H_2O?**

$$H_2O\ (g) \rightarrow H_2\ (g) + \frac{1}{2} O_2\ (g) \qquad H = {}^+57.8\ \textbf{kj/mole}$$

⁻57.8 kj/mole

❑❑ **What is Hess's law of summation?**

If two or more chemical reactions are combined by subtraction or addition to form a final product, then subtracting or adding the enthalpies in the same fashion will give the change in enthalpy of the reaction. These calculations are able to be performed since enthalpy is a function of state, not pathway.

❑❑ **What is entropy?**

Entropy is a measure of the *DISORDER* of a system. The higher the entropy, the greater the disorder. Thus, used in a sentence, one might say "Mike Donnino's office exhibits a great deal of entropy." Entropy is symbolized by the letter S.

❑❑ **What sign (positive or negative) indicates increased disorder?**

The *more positive,* the greater the *disorder.*

❑❑ **Place the following in order of lowest to highest entropy:**

Solid, Liquid, Gas

Solid (least disorder) → liquid → gas

❑❑ **How do you calculate the change in entropy?**

$\Delta S = S_{final} - S_{initial}$. Since entropy is a state function, it depends only on the final and initial states.

❑❑ **What is the second law of thermodynamics?**

The second law of thermodynamics states that every chemical process increases the entropy of the universe.

❑❑ **What does it mean for a reaction to be "spontaneous"?**

Practically speaking, a spontaneous reaction is one that proceeds *from LEFT to RIGHT*.

❑❑ **What parameter determines if a reaction is spontaneous or not?**

If your answer is enthalpy, then you have the company of many of the early scientists. But, as they discovered, some reactions are spontaneous but are endothermic. Thus, this is incorrect.

If you think entropy is the answer, you are technically correct, BUT this probably will not help you on the MCAT. The entropy of the UNIVERSE always increases in a chemical process (i.e., second law of thermodynamics). If the entropy of the universe increases, then the reaction is spontaneous. Unfortunately, "scientist Bob" cannot constantly be measuring the entropy of the entire universe (system + surroundings).

Luckily, a state property exists which can determine if a reaction is spontaneous or not by measuring the entropy and enthalpy of the SYSTEM without having to take into account the surroundings. The property is termed *GIBBS FREE ENERGY (G)* and is defined as follows:

$\Delta G = \Delta H - T\Delta S$

$\Delta G < 0$ → Spontaneous (goes toward the right)
$\Delta G = 0$ → Equilibrium
$\Delta G > 0$ → Non-spontaneous (goes toward the left)

<u>Bottom Line</u>: *Memorize the formula for Gibbs free energy* and the criteria that follow in order to determine if a reaction is spontaneous.   At the same time, understand that the entropy of the universe (system + surroundings) will also be a determinate of spontaneous reactions.

❑❑ **T/F: If the enthalpy of a reaction is negative and the entropy is positive, then the reaction is spontaneous.**

True. Manipulate the formula for Gibbs free energy ($\Delta G = \Delta H - T\Delta S$) to see why this is so. Plug any negative enthalpy combined with any positive entropy into the equation and you will see that the result is always a negative number.

❏❏ **T/F: If the enthalpy of a reaction is positive and the entropy is negative, then the reaction is spontaneous.**

False. The reaction is non-spontaneous. Again, manipulate the formula for Gibbs free energy to see why this is so.

❏❏ **If the enthalpy of a reaction is positive and the entropy is positive, what determines if a reaction is spontaneous or not?**

Temperature. Again, use the Gibbs free energy equation to understand this concept. The temperature multiplied by the entropy must be greater than the enthalpy for the Gibbs free energy to be negative. Thus, high temperatures make these types of reactions spontaneous.

❏❏ **Fill in the chart:**

Enthalpy (ΔH)	Entropy (ΔS)	Gibbs Free Energy (ΔG)	? Spontaneous
+	-		
-	+		
+	+		
-	-		

Enthalpy (ΔH)	Entropy (ΔS)	Gibbs Free Energy (ΔG)	? Spontaneous
+	-	+	No
-	+	-	Yes
+	+	+/-	At high temperatures
-	-	+/-	At low temperatures

❏❏ **Predict the sign of the enthalpy change in the following:**

$$H_2O \ (g) \rightarrow H_2O \ (s)$$

Negative. In going from gas to solid, entropy decreases (S < 0). Thus, in order for the reaction to be able to occur, enthalpy must be negative (H < 0).

❏❏ **What is an exergonic reaction? Endergonic reaction?**

An exergonic reaction is a spontaneous reaction (G < 0), whereas an endergonic reaction is a non-spontaneous reaction (G > 0).

❏❏ **What is the relationship between Gibbs free energy (ΔG) and the equilibrium constant (K) ?**

$\Delta G = -RT\ln K$

Equilibrium: $\Delta G = 0$ $K = 1$

Spontaneous: $\Delta G < 0$ $K > 1$

Non-spontaneous: $\Delta G > 0$ $K < 1$

Simply stated:
If ΔG is negative, K>1
If ΔG is positive, K<1
If ΔG=0, K=1

❏❏ **T/F: The lower the ΔG (more negative), the faster the reaction.**

False! Remember that thermodynamics and kinetics of a reaction are separate concepts. Thus, the value of ΔG has no impact on the speed of a reaction.

❏❏ **What is the ΔG for the following reaction? Is the reaction spontaneous or non-spontaneous?**

$$H_2 + Cl_2 \rightarrow 2\ HCl \quad \Delta H = -92\ kj/mole$$
$$\Delta S = {}^+186\ J/K\ mol$$
$$T = 25^\circ\ Celsius$$

$\Delta G = -97$ kj/mol. Use the formula, $\Delta G = \Delta H - T\Delta S$. Remember to convert entropy to kilojoules in order to calculate!! Since ΔG is negative, the reaction is spontaneous. Note that in this equation, the negative sign of ΔG could be determined based on the negative enthalpy and positive entropy.

ACIDS AND BASES

❑❑ **What is an Arrhenius acid?**

Arrhenius acid: Any compound that releases H^+ when added to an *aqueous* solution.

Example: $^*HCl + H_2O \rightarrow H_3O^+ + Cl^-$

❑❑ **What is an Arrhenius base?**

Arrhenius base: Any compound that forms OH^- when added to an *aqueous* solution.

Example: $^*NaOH + H_2O \rightarrow {}^-OH + Na^+$

❑❑ **What is a Brønsted-Lowry acid?**

Brønsted-Lowry acid: Any compound that *DONATES* a *proton* (hydrogen).

Example: $^*HCl + NaOH \rightarrow H_2O + NaCl$

❑❑ **What is a Brønsted-Lowry base?**

Brønsted-Lowry base: Any compound that *ACCEPTS* a *proton* (hydrogen).

Example: $HCl + {}^*NaOH \rightarrow H_2O + NaCl$

❑❑ **What is a Lewis acid?**

Lewis acid: A chemical species that *accepts* a pair of *electrons* from another chemical species.

Example: $^*BF_3 + F^- \rightarrow BF_4^-$

❑❑ **What is a Lewis base?**

Lewis base: A chemical species that *donates* a pair of *electrons* to another chemical species.

Example: $BF_3 + {}^*F^- \rightarrow BF_4^-$

❑❑   **T/F: A Lewis acid is, by definition, an Arrhenius acid.**

False. Note in the above definition and example that the Lewis acid does not form H_3O^+.
An Arrhenius acid is a compound that forms H^+ when added to an aqueous solution.
Thus, a Lewis acid is not necessarily an Arrhenius acid.

❑❑   **T/F: An Arrhenius acid is, by definition, a Lewis acid.**

True. Arrhenius maintained a narrow definition of acid (i.e., formation of H_3O^+).
Brønsted expanded on this definition to include all hydrogen donors whether or not H^+
formed as product. Lewis further expanded the definition to include all electron
acceptors. Thus, the three definitions are arranged from specific (i.e., Arrhenius) to
general (i.e., Lewis). The Lewis acid is the most general definition, and all Arrhenius
acids are by definition Lewis acids as well.

❑❑   **What is the "K_a?" Use the following equation to define and explain.**

$$HCl + H_2O \text{ (aq)} \rightarrow H_3O^+ + Cl^-$$

The K_a is the equilibrium expression for an acid. Remember, solids and liquids do not
factor into the equilibrium equation. Thus, the K_a for the above equation would be:

$K_a = [H_3O^+][Cl^-]/[HCl]$

❑❑   **Which is more acidic: K_a=1.5 or K_a=2?**

The higher the K_a, the more acidic. Thus, $K_a = 2$ is more acidic. For example, the
chemical equation in the previous question was:

$HCl + H_2O \text{ (aq)} \rightarrow H_3O^+ + Cl^-$

$K_a = [H_3O^+][Cl^-]/[HCl]$

Since the stronger acid dissociates more, this will yield a larger amount of H_3O^+ and a
smaller of amount of HCl. As can be seen from the equilibrium expression, this will
create a larger K_a.

❑❑   **What does pK_a mean?**

Remember that p means "*negative log*." Thus, $pK_a = ^- log [K_a]$. This conversion allows
the K_a of an equation to be defined by a manageable number, the pK_a.

❑❑   **Which is more acidic: pK_a=1 or pK_a=2?**

The lower the pK_a, the more acidic. Thus, pK_a=1 is more acidic.

❑❑ **What does pH mean?**

Again, p means "negative log." Thus, pH = $^-$log [hydrogen ions].

❑❑ **Why bother converting hydrogen ions into pH?**

Converting from hydrogen ions into pH allows for conversion into a more easily managed number. For example, a H^+ concentration equal to 1.0×10^{-7} equals a pH of 7.

❑❑ **Which is more acidic: a solution with pH=5 or pH=6?**

The lower the pH, the more acidic the solution. Thus, pH=5 is more acidic.

❑❑ **What is the pH of a neutral solution? An acidic solution? Basic solution?**

Neutral → pH = 7
Acidic → pH < 7
Basic → pH > 7

❑❑ **What is the self-ionization of water?**

Water (H_2O) so-called "self-ionizes" in the following manner:

$$H_2O \text{ (l)} + H_2O \text{ (l)} \rightarrow H_3O^+ \text{ (aq)} + OH^- \text{ (aq)}$$

In this fashion, one water molecule acts as the acid and the other water molecule acts as the base. In the face of a strong acid or base, this self-ionization of water is often negligible.

❑❑ **What is the equilibrium expression for the self-ionization of water? See previous equation.**

$K_w = [H_3O^+][OH^-]$. Remember, *liquid* is *not* factored into the equilibrium equation.

❑❑ **What is the definition of K_w?**

K_w is a measure of the tendency of water to dissociate into H^+ and ^-OH. Although K_w is set up as an equilibrium expression, H_2O (l) is not factored into the equation since it is liquid. Thus, the K_w is similar to the K_{sp} (ion-product constant) in that it is dependent only on the products.

$$K_w = [H^+][OH^-] = 10^{-14}$$

❑❑ **The pH of an aqueous solution is 5. What is the pOH of this solution?**

The pOH =9. The *total* of pH and pOH of an aqueous solution is always *14*.
Thus, pH + pOH = 14. Hence, 14 − 5 = 9.

❏❏ **What is the K_b?**

K_b is the equilibrium expression for a base.

❏❏ **The K_b of A is 1.3 whereas the K_b of B is 1.7. Which (A or B) is the stronger base?**

B is a stronger base than A. The larger the K_b, the stronger the base. This is similar to K_a in that the higher the K_a, the stronger the acid.

❏❏ **Compound A has a pK_b of 3. Compound B has a pK_b of 4. Which is the stronger base?**

Compound A is the stronger base. The lower the pK_b, the stronger the base. This again is similar to the pK_a in that the lower the pK_a, the stronger the acid.

❏❏ **What is the conjugate base of CH_3COOH in the following reaction?**

$$CH_3COOH \longleftrightarrow CH_3COO^- + H^+$$

The conjugate base of CH_3COOH is CH_3COO^-. The conjugate base is formed when the acid (CH_3COOH) gives up a hydrogen and forms a base (CH_3COO^-). In a similar fashion, CH_3COOH is the conjugate acid of CH_3COO^-.

❏❏ **Label the following as acid or base and match up the conjugate acid/base pairs.**

$$HCl + H_2O \rightarrow H_3O^+ + {}^-Cl$$

$HCl + H_2O \rightarrow H_3O^+ + {}^-Cl$
Acid   Base   Acid   Base

HCl (conjugate acid) of ^-Cl (conjugate base)
H_2O (conjugate base) of H_3O^+ (conjugate acid)

❏❏ **What value results from multiplying K_a x K_b of a conjugate acid/base pair?**

$K_w = K_aK_b$ for a conjugate acid/base pair.

❏❏ **What are some examples of strong acids?**

Strong acids: HCl, H_2SO_4, HI, HNO_3, HBr, $HClO_4$

❏❏ **What are some examples of strong bases?**

Strong bases: $NaOH$, $LiOH$, KOH

❑❑ **T/F: A strong acid is fully dissociated in solution.**

True.

❑❑ **What does it mean to say a compound such as a strong acid is "fully dissociated"?**

This can best be explained by an example. HCl is a strong acid. If HCl is placed in an aqueous solution, it will form almost 100% H^+ and Cl^-. Thus, the hydrogen and the chloride will be "fully dissociated" from each other.

$HCl \rightarrow H^+ + Cl^-$

❑❑ **Is a strong base fully dissociated in solution as well?**

Yes.

❑❑ **Is acetic acid (shown below) a weak or a strong acid?**

$$CH_3COOH$$

Acetic acid is a weak acid.

❑❑ **Is a weak acid fully dissociated in a solution?**

No. On the contrary, only a very small percentage of the weak acid dissociates in solution. For example, if CH_3COOH is placed in an aqueous solution, less than 2% will dissociate to form CH_3COO^- and H^+.

$CH_3COOH \rightarrow CH_3COO^- + H^+$

❑❑ **What is the pH of a solution of .1 M of HCl? How is this calculated? Is HCl a strong or weak acid and does this factor into the determination of the pH?**

HCl is a strong acid and therefore is completely dissociated in solution. Thus, .1 M (100%) of H^+ is formed.

$pH = {}^-log\,[H^+] \rightarrow pH = {}^-log_{10}\,(.1) \rightarrow pH = {}^-log_{10}\,(1 \times 10^{-1}) \rightarrow {}^-(-1.0) \rightarrow 1.0$

Thus, pH = 1.

❑❑ **A solution of HCl has a pH of 5.0. What is the H_3O^+ (aq) concentration?**

Since HCl is a strong acid, it fully dissociates in solution. This allows for the calculation of hydrogen ion concentration:
$pH = {}^-log\,[H^+] \rightarrow 5 = {}^-log\,[H^+] \rightarrow 5 = {}^-log_{10}\,(1 \times 10^{-5})$. Thus, $[H^+] = 1 \times 10^{-5}$.

❏❏   **A solution of CH$_3$COOH has a pH of 5.0. What is the H$_3$0$^+$ (aq) concentration?**

Unfortunately, this cannot be solved as easily as the previous question. CH$_3$COOH is a weak acid and does not fully dissociate in solution. Therefore, more information would be needed to calculate this answer.

❏❏   **What is an amphoteric species?**

An amphoteric substance can act as either an acid or a base, depending on the chemical environment. For example, water can act as either an acid or a base, depending on the circumstances of the reaction.

BUFFERS

❏❏ **Match the following titration curves:**

Titration of a strong acid with .10 M NaOH
Titration of a weak acid with .10 M NaOH

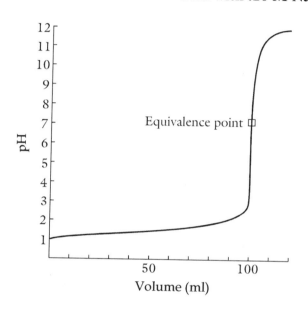 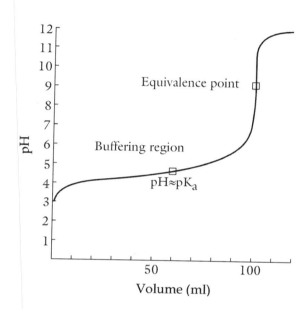

The graph on the left illustrates the titration of a strong acid and a strong base, whereas the graph on the right shows the titration of a weak acid and a strong base. Notice the difference in the curves and the different pH at each starting point.

❏❏ **What are two characteristics of a good buffer?**

Two characteristics of a good buffer:

1. Composed of weak base/acid.
2. The pH and pK_a are relatively equal.

❏❏ **Should a good buffer be composed of a large or small amount of weak acid/base?**

A large amount. The increased amount of BOTH weak acid and weak base can more readily compensate for the addition of more acid or base.

❏❏ What is the equivalence point of a buffer?

This is the point at which the TOTAL amount of chemical acid and chemical base are equal. DO NOT confuse this with the point where concentration of the weak acid and weak base making up the buffer are equal. This is a very common mistake. In the example below, you can see that the equivalence point is much past the point where $CH_3COOH = CH_3COO^-$ (i.e., pH = pK_a).

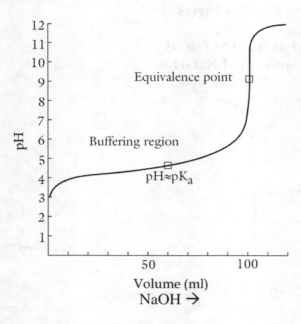

This curve represents titration of CH_3COOH (weak acid) with NaOH (strong base).

❏❏ What is the buffer zone?

As noted on the graph in the previous question, the buffer zone is the region where pH remains essentially constant despite increases in the volume of acid added to the solution.

❏❏ State the Henderson-Hasselbalch equation.

pH= pK_a + log base/acid.

❏❏ What are the implications of the Henderson-Hasselbalch equation?

When the amount of conjugate base = conjugate acid, the pH of the solution equals the pK_a of the solution.

❏❏ The pH of a buffer solution is 3.78 when the weak base and the conjugate acid of the buffer are equivalent. What is the pK_a of this solution?

Apply the Henderson-Hasselbalch equation: pH=pK_a + log base/acid.

Thus, when base=acid, log base/acid = log 1.

The log of 1 equals 0.

Thus, $pH=pK_a$...therefore $pK_a=3.78$.

The point of this question is to keep in mind that when the acid and the base that make up a buffer are equal, then the $pH=pK_a$!!

❑❑ **What are some examples of buffers in the human body?**

Examples of intracellular buffers are phosphates and cytosolic proteins. The main extracellular buffer is the CO_2/HCO_3^- system given below:

$$CO_2 + H_2O \leftrightarrow H_2CO_3 \leftrightarrow HCO_3^- + H^+$$

❑❑ **What is the normal range of pH that our body buffers struggle to maintain?**

In the normal state, these buffers function to keep our body pH in the range of 7.35-7.45. This tight control of our body pH is essential to our well-being.

GASES

❑❑ **What is a gas?**

A gas is a state of matter in which the atoms are in constant, rapid motion and spread a great distance apart relative to their small size. Gases conform to the shape of their container and will fill the container uniformly.

❑❑ **What are four parameters used to describe a gas?**

Volume, pressure, temperature, and quantity.

❑❑ **How does a gas cause pressure?**

The atoms that compose a gas collide against each other and the walls of the container. These collisions against the walls of the container result in pressure.

❑❑ **What units are used to describe pressure of a gas? What is their relationship?**

1 atmosphere = 760 mmHg = 760 torr.

❑❑ **What is the difference between an ideal and a real gas?**

Both an ideal gas and a real gas consist of atoms in constant motion. In an ideal gas (theoretical) the attractive and repulsive forces between these atoms are negligible, but in reality (i.e., real gas) attractive forces do exist.

❑❑ **What are the attractive/repulsive forces between atoms in real gases called?**

These attractive/repulsive forces are termed van der Waals forces.

❑❑ **In an ideal gas, are collisions between particles elastic or non-elastic?**

Collisions are elastic, meaning that there is no loss of energy from friction.

❑❑ **Is a gas without volume an ideal or a real gas?**

An ideal gas has no volume.

❑❑ **Are van der Waals forces weak or strong?**

These are very *weak* forces.

❑❑ **Van der Waals proposed an equation to account for the attractive forces between molecules. Do I have to know the van der Waals equation (noted below)?**

$$(p + an^2/V^2)\ (V- nb) = nRT$$

Ideally, you will not be asked to reproduce this complicated equation. If a calculation is called for, the formula should be provided for you. Note that an^2/V^2 accounts for intermolecular forces, and nb represents the volume of the non-ideal gas molecules.

❑❑ **What conditions cause the greatest deviation from the ideal gas law? In other words, when do van der Waals forces affect gases the most?**

At very *low temperatures* (i.e., decreased kinetic energy) and very *high pressures* (i.e., molecules are in close contact), van der Waals forces have the most influence on the gas.

❑❑ **Which is more likely to follow the ideal gas law, a low density gas or a high density gas?**

A *low density* gas is more likely to follow the ideal gas law because decreased density implies decreased van der Waals (attractive/repulsive) forces.

❑❑ **What is "STP"?**

Standard temperature and pressure. This is defined as:
- Temperature = 273° Kelvin or O° Celsius
- Pressure = 760 mmHG or 1 atm or 760 torr

❑❑ **Convert 30° Celsius into Kelvin.**

T (Kelvin) = 273 + t (Celsius). Thus, 273 + 30 = *303° Kelvin*.

❑❑ **What is absolute zero?**

The Kelvin scale of temperature begins at zero. This is the absolute lowest limit that temperature can reach. The Celsius equivalent is ⁻273°.

❑❑ **How much volume does 1 mole of gas occupy at STP?**

22.4 liters.

❑❑ **What is a standard molar volume?**

A standard molar volume is the volume that 1 mole of gas occupies at STP. As noted in the previous question, this equals 22.4 liters.

❑❑ **What is Boyle's law?**

Boyle's law states that at constant temperature the volume of a fixed amount of gas is inversely proportional to the pressure. Thus,

Volume = 1/pressure and PV = k (constant) or $P_1V_1 = P_2V_2$

❑❑ **What is Charles' law?**

Charles' law states that at constant pressure the volume of a fixed amount of an ideal gas is directly proportional to its absolute temperature. Thus,

Volume = Temperature and V/T = k or $V_1/T_1 = V_2/T_2$

❑❑ **What is the ideal gas law (i.e., the formula)?**

$PV=nRT$ where

P = pressure, V = volume, n = number of moles, R = constant, T = temperature

❑❑ **What is another form of the ideal gas law, sometimes termed the combined gas law?**

$P_1V_1/T_1 = P_2V_2/T_2$

❑❑ **I am tired of all these laws! Do I really need to know all of them?**

Actually, by memorizing and understanding the ideal gas law (PV=nRT), all of these other formulas can be quickly derived. Simple algebra allows you to say:

PV/nRT = k (constant)

Thus, $P_1V_1/T_1 = P_2V_2/T_2$ (n and R are constant and cancel out – i.e., combined gas law).
Also, $P_1V_1 = P_2V_2$ (when temperature is constant, cancel it out – i.e., Boyle's law).
And, $V_1/T_1 = V_2/P_2$ (when pressure is constant, cancel it out – i.e., Charles' law).

❑❑ **How many moles of carbon would be present in a volume of gas of 44.8 liters at STP?**

44.8 liters x 1 mole of carbon/22.4 liters = 2 moles of carbon.

❑❑ **What is Dalton's law of partial pressures of gases?**

The total pressure of a gas is equal to the sum of the partial pressures of the components of that gas.

Pressure $_{(total)}$ = $P_a + P_b + P_c$

❑❑   **What formula relates the total pressure, fractional percent, and partial pressure of a gas?**

The total pressure multiplied by fractional percent of a gas equals the partial pressure of that gas. That is,
Pressure $_{(total)}$ (fraction or percent of P_a) = P_a

❑❑   **How do you calculate the mole fraction?**

Mole fraction = $\dfrac{\text{\# of moles of X}}{\text{Total \# of moles}}$

❑❑   **Flashback question: How do you calculate the number of moles of a given substance?**

Number of moles = $\dfrac{\text{Weight of sample (grams)}}{\text{Molecular weight (grams/mole)}}$

❑❑   **A gaseous mixture contains .3 moles of oxygen, .6 moles of carbon dioxide, and .3 moles of nitrogen. The total pressure in the system is 400 mmHg. What is the partial pressure of carbon dioxide? Oxygen? Nitrogen?**

This question requires knowledge of Dalton's law of partial pressures.
First, calculate the total moles of gaseous mixture: .3 + .6 + .3 = 1.2
Then calculate the mole fraction of CO_2:

Mole fraction of CO_2 = moles of CO_2 / total moles of gas
                          = .6 / 1.2 = .5

Partial pressure of CO_2 = (mole fraction of CO_2) x (total pressure)
                           = (.5) x (400 mmHg)
                           = 200 mmHg

Mole fraction of O_2 = moles of O_2 / total moles of gas
                          = .3 / 1.2 = .25

Partial pressure of O_2 = (mole fraction of O_2) x (total pressure)
                           = (.25) x (400 mmHg)
                           = 100 mmHg

Nitrogen → see oxygen above (i.e., same calculations)

❑❑ **What is the partial pressure of oxygen in the oral cavity during inhalation?**

Pressure $_{(total)}$ = 760mmHg
Recall from biology that the oxygen present in atmosphere = 21% or .21
Thus,

Pressure $_{(total)}$ (fractional coefficient or percent of $P_{(oxygen)}$) = $P_{(oxygen)}$
760 mmHg X .21 = 160 mmHg

❑❑ **After the following reaction is run to completion, the pressure is recorded as 1.2 atmospheres. What is the partial pressure of N_2 (g)?**

$$2NH_3 (g) \rightarrow N_2(g) + 3 H_2 (g)$$

The total moles of gas of the products of the complete reaction = 4. The total pressure is 1.2 atmospheres. 1.2/4 = .3. Thus, each mole exerts .3 atmospheres of pressure to make the total of 1.2 atmospheres. Since there is only one N_2 (g), the partial pressure of N_2 (g) = .3 atmospheres.

❑❑ **A patient in the intensive care unit is on a ventilator system. Each volume of air that the system delivers is set at a constant 700 ml. The pressure in the system is initially recorded at 20 cmH_2O. If the tidal volume (volume of air delivered) is decreased to 500 ml, what would you expect the pressure to be?**

Remember, $P_1 V_1 = P_2 V_2$ (see earlier question for a way to quickly derive this from PV = nrt.)

Thus, (20 cm H_2O) (700 ml) = (X cm H_2O) (500 ml)

28 = X cm H_2O; Thus, 28 cm H_2O

❑❑ **T/F: The density of a gas is directly related to the pressure and molar mass of a gas.**

True.

❑❑ **As noted, the density of a gas is directly related to pressure and molar mass of a gas. State this in a complete formula.**

Density = $\dfrac{P \times M}{RT}$ where P = pressure, M= molar mass, R = gas constant, T = temp.

❑❑ **What is Graham's law of effusion?**

Graham's law of effusion states that the ratio of effusion of two gases is inversely proportional to the ratio of the molecular weights of these two gases.

❏❏ **State Graham's law of effusion in a formula:**

R1/R2 = [M2/M1] ^{½}

R1 = Rate of effusion of gas #1
R2 = Rate of effusion of gas #2
M1 = Molecular weight of gas #1
M2 = Molecular weight of gas #2

KINETICS

❑❑ **What is the rate law of the following reaction?**

$$2A + B_2 \rightarrow 3C + D$$

This is a trick question. The rate law must be determined *experimentally*. Thus, without knowing more information you cannot answer this question. The rate law would be the concentration of the reacting molecules (i.e., A and B) raised to an experimentally determined power. The only exception is if the reaction is an elementary reaction.

❑❑ **What is an elementary reaction?**

An elementary reaction is one that has no intermediates or additional steps needed to form products. An "overall reaction" (which is typically what you are given) is made up of a series of "elementary" reactions. As noted previously, a rate law can be known from the equation *only* if the reaction is elementary. Otherwise, the rate law must be known experimentally or deduced from the series of elementary reactions that make up the reaction in question.

❑❑ **Determine the rate law based on the experimental data:**

$$X + Y \rightarrow Z$$

Experiment	Concentration of X (M)	Concentration of Y (M)	Rate of reaction (M/sec)
1	0.1	0.1	2×10^{-2}
2	0.2	0.1	8×10^{-2}
3	0.1	0.2	2×10^{-2}

Rate = $k [X]^2$. As you can see, as the concentration of X doubled, the rate of the reaction quadrupled. In contrast, as the concentration of Y doubled, the rate remained the same. Thus, the concentration of Y is not a factor in the rate law and X should be squared in order to get quadruple the rate.

❑❑ **What is the rate law of the following reaction?**

$$C_2H_6 \text{ (g)} \rightarrow 2 CH_3$$

Again, the rate law must be determined experimentally. The actual rate law of this reaction is rate = $k [C_2H_6]^2$. This question illustrates the need for experimental determination of the rate law, as the coefficient in the reaction does not correlate with the power to which C_2H_6 is raised.

❑❑ **What is the rate constant?**

The rate constant k was defined by Arrhenius in 1887 as follows:

$k = A e^{-Ea/RT}$ where Ea is energy per mole, R = gas constant.

❑❑ **Does the rate law vary in regard to temperature?**

Yes. As noted in the formula in the previous question, the rate of reaction increases with increase in temperature. Exact determinations can be made by applying the formula, but a general estimate is that for every 10 degree rise in temperature, the reaction rate doubles.

❑❑ **What is a reaction intermediate?**

This is a chemical species that is formed during a reaction for a brief period. The reaction intermediate is formed and consumed in the reaction and does not appear in the overall reaction equation.

❑❑ **What is a catalyst?**

A catalyst is a substance that *speeds* a chemical reaction.

❑❑ **Is a catalyst consumed in the reaction?**

No. A catalyst is not consumed or changed in a chemical reaction.

❑❑ **How does a catalyst speed a chemical reaction?**

A catalyst *lowers the activation energy* needed for the reaction to proceed. Note that the catalyst lowers the activation energy for both the forward and the backward reactions.

❑❑ **Which way will a catalyst speed the following reaction?**

$$A + B \longleftrightarrow C + D$$

This is another trick question. Remember, a catalyst will *not* determine which way the reaction proceeds. A catalyst will speed *both* sides of the reaction, bringing the reaction toward equilibrium faster. Recall that the thermodynamics of a reaction, NOT THE KINETICS, determines the direction in which the reaction proceeds or where the equilibrium lies. In other words, a *catalyst does not affect the thermodynamics of a reaction.*

❑❑ **What are biological catalysts called? What type of substance are they?**

Enzymes. With rare exceptions, enzymes are *proteins*.

❏❏ How is the rate order determined from a *known* rate law?

The rate order is determined by adding the superscripts of the rate law.

❏❏ What is the rate order of the following experimentally determined rate law?

$$\text{Rate} = k\,[HCl]^2\,[H_2O]^1$$

This is a *third-order* reaction. This is determined by adding the superscripts of the rate law. Thus, $2 + 1 = 3$.

❏❏ Is there such an entity as a zero-order reaction? If yes, explain.

Yes. A zero-order reaction does not depend on concentration of reactants. Instead, the rate constant alone determines the rate of reaction. Thus,

$\text{Rate} = k$

❏❏ What can be said of half-life in a first-order reaction?

In a first-order reaction, a graph of the natural logarithm of the concentration against time is a straight line. From this straight line, the rate constant can be calculated and related to the half-life of a substance. The half-life ($t_{1/2}$) is the time it takes for a substance to fall to one-half of its original value. The following formula relates half-life with the rate constant.

$t_{1/2} = \,^{-}\ln_{1/2}/k = .693/k$

❏❏ What is meant by kinetic versus thermodynamic control of a reaction?

Reactions often can form more than one product. In these cases, the products are often affected by the reaction conditions. The kinetic control of a reaction refers to when the favored products are those that form at a greater rate. The thermodynamic control of the reaction refers to when the favored products are those that are formed based on lowest energy.

❏❏ What conditions favor the kinetic control of a reaction?

Conditions that favor kinetic control of a reaction are low temperatures and short reaction times.

❏❏ What conditions favor thermodynamic control of a reaction?

Conditions that favor thermodynamic control of a reaction are high temperatures and long reaction times.

PHASE AND SOLUTION CHEMISTRY

❑❑ **What is the difference between solid, liquid, and gas?**

Solid is a phase of matter that has definite shape and volume. Liquid has volume but no definite shape. Gas has neither definite shape nor volume.

❑❑ **What is the triple point?**

The triple point is the point at which the three phases of matter co-exist in equilibrium. This occurs at a specific temperature and pressure.

❑❑ **What is a solution?**

A solution is a homogenous system that contains two or more substances.

❑❑ **What is the difference between a solute and a solvent?**

A solvent is typically the major component of a solution and a solute is the minor component of a solution. This distinction is hard to make at times.

❑❑ **What is a miscible solution?**

Two solutions that when mixed together form a one-phase solution.

❑❑ **What two types of solutions will form a miscible solution?**

Two polar solutions or two non-polar solutions will form miscible solutions. Remember that "like dissolves like".

❑❑ **What is a immiscible solution?**

Two solutions which form a two-phase solution when mixed.

❑❑ **What are the two types of solutions that would form an immiscible solution?**

A polar solution mixed with a non-polar solution.

❑❑   **What is molarity?**

Molarity is defined as the number of moles per liter of solution.

❑❑   **What is molality?**

Molality is defined as the number of moles per kilogram of solvent.

❑❑   **Does temperature affect molarity or molality? Why?**

Temperature affects molarity but not molality. Temperature affects volume which in turn affects the molarity since it is defined per *liter* of solution.

❑❑   **What is normality?**

Normality is defined as the number of equivalents of either acid or base.

❑❑   **What is the normality of H_2SO_4?**

Normality = 2. There are two equivalents of acid – "H_2".

❑❑   **What is a colligative property?**

A colligative property is one that applies to a solution based on the number of solute particles without regard to the particular identity of the solution.

❑❑   **Name four key colligative properties.**

Vapor pressure lowering, boiling point elevation, freezing point depression, and osmotic pressure.

❑❑   **What is vapor pressure lowering?**

When a solute is dissolved in a solvent, the vapor pressure of the solution is lower than the vapor pressure of the pure solvent.

❑❑   **What is the formula for determining the vapor pressure lowering of a solution?**

P $= X_B P_A^{\,o}$
P   = change in vapor pressure of the solution
X_B = mole fraction of the solute
$P_A^{\,o}$ = vapor pressure of the pure solvent

❑❑   **What is boiling point elevation?**

When a solute is added to a solution, the boiling point of that solution is elevated.

❏❏ **What is the formula for determining the boiling point elevation?**

T_b = ik_bm
T_b = boiling point elevation
i = number of particles the solute dissociates into
k_b = constant ($C°kg/mol$)
m = molality

❏❏ **As winter approaches, you add antifreeze to the radiator of your car. What principle of chemistry did you employ in order to prevent the water in the radiator from freezing?**

Freezing point depression.

❏❏ **What is freezing point depression?**

When a solute is added to a solution, the freezing point of that solution is decreased.

❏❏ **What is the formula for freezing point depression?**

T_f = ik_fm
i = number of particles into which solute dissolves into solvent
k_f = freezing point constant
m = molality of the solution

❏❏ **What is osmotic pressure?**

Osmotic pressure is the pressure that would need to be applied to a solution to prevent molecules from diffusing through a semi-permeable membrane.

❏❏ **What is the formula for osmotic pressure?**

Osmotic pressure = $(n/V)RT = MRT$
n = number of moles of solute
V = solution volume (liters)
R = gas constant
T = Kelvin temperature
M = n/V or molar concentration of solute

❏❏ **What is K_{sp}?**

The K_{sp} is an equilibrium constant for the dissolution of a soluble solid. "sp" stands for the solubility constant.

❏❏ **What is the K$_{sp}$ of the following solution:**

$$AgCl \text{ (s)} \rightleftharpoons Ag + \text{(aq)} + Cl^{-}\text{(aq)}$$

$K_{sp} = [Ag^{+}][Cl]$.

❏❏ **What is the calculated ion product (Q)?**

The calculated ion product is the product of the solute and the solvent just after mixing but *before* a reaction takes place.

❏❏ **How can you determine if a precipitation will occur?**

Compare the ion product of the solution (Q) with the established K_{sp}.   If the $Q > K_{sp}$, then the solute precipitates. If $Q < K_{sp}$, then the solute dissolves.

❏❏ **T/F: The higher the K$_{sp}$, the more soluble the compound.**

True.

❏❏ **What is the common ion effect?**

The common ion effect refers to the decreased solubility of a salt when an ion of that salt is already present in solution. For example, AgCl would have a lower solubility when immersed in a solution of NaCl and H_2O. Chloride is the "common ion" which causes the decreased solubility.

ELECTROCHEMISTRY

❏❏ **What is an anion?**

An anion is a negatively charged ion.

❏❏ **What is a cation?**

A cation is a positively charged ion.

❏❏ **What is oxidation?**

Oxidation is a loss of electrons.

❏❏ **What is reduction?**

Reduction is a gain of electrons.

❏❏ **What is the difference between oxidation and an oxidizing agent? What is the difference between reduction and a reducing agent?**

This is a concept that is often confused. An "oxidizing agent" allows for the oxidation of another substance. Thus, the *oxidizing agent itself is reduced,* not oxidized. Likewise, a "reducing agent" allows for the reduction of another substance. Thus, the *reducing agent itself is oxidized.*

❏❏ **What is the electric potential (ΔE)?**

Electric potential is the potential electrical difference between two charged half-cells.

❏❏ **What is the definition of electrical work (W_{elec}) (i.e., formula)?**

$W_{elec} = -Q\,E$

❏❏ **What is the relationship between free energy (ΔG) and W_{elec}?**

At constant temperature and pressure in a galvanic cell, $\Delta G = W_{elec}$. Thus, $\Delta G = -Q\,E$

❏❏ **Where does reduction take place – anode or cathode?**

Reduction takes place at the *cathode.* Remember, "*Red Cat.*"

❑❑ **Where does oxidation take place – anode or cathode?**

Oxidation takes place at the anode.

❑❑ **What is the difference between a galvanic and an electrolytic cell?**

In a *galvanic* cell, the two half-cell substances reactant *spontaneously*. The E is positive. In an *electrolytic* cell, the reaction is *non-spontaneous* and requires the input of electricity in order to propel the reaction. E is negative in this case.

❑❑ **Two half-cells are combined to make a galvanic cell. Reduction takes place at which half-cell?**

Reduction takes place at the half-cell with the *more positive* reduction potential (E^o).

❑❑ **What is the formula used to determine the standard half-cell reduction potential (ΔE^o)?**

$\Delta E^o = E^o$ (cathode) $- E^o$ (anode)

❑❑ **Bromide and hydrogen are both half-cells with the following reduction potentials. If connected in a galvanic cell, which would be reduced/oxidized? What is the ΔE?**

$$Br_2 + 2e^- \rightarrow 2\,Br^- \quad 1.065$$
$$2H^+ + 2e^- \rightarrow H_2 \quad 0$$

Br_2 will be reduced and H^+ will be oxidized because Br_2 has the more positive reduction potential. Recall, $\Delta E^o = E^o$ (cathode) $- E^o$ (anode). Thus, $1.065 - 0 = 1.065$

❑❑ **What is the relationship between ΔG and ΔE?**

$\Delta G = -nF\Delta E$ where n is the number of moles of electrons and F is Faraday's constant.

❑❑ **When ΔE is negative, what sign will ΔG have?**

When ΔE is negative, ΔG will be positive. When ΔE is positive, ΔG will be negative.

❑❑ **T/F: The larger the negative E, the stronger the reducing agent.**

True.

❑❑ **T/F: The larger the positive E, the stronger the oxidizing agent.**

True.

❑❑ **What is Faraday's first law?**

Faraday's first law (paraphrased) states that the quantities of substance produced or consumed at the electrodes of a cell are proportional to the amount of electrical charge that passes through the cell.

❑❑ **What is Faraday's second law?**

Faraday's second law (paraphrased) states that the quantity of a substance produced or consumed at the electrodes of a cell is proportional to its molar mass divided by the number of electrons transferred per formula unit.

❑❑ **T/F: Non-metals have low electrical conductivity.**

True.

❑❑ **T/F: I am tired of doing chemistry.**

True. If you answered false, consider taking GRE instead of MCAT and pursue a chemistry career.

ORGANIC CHEMISTRY

HYDROCARBONS (ALKANES, ALKENES AND ALKYNES)

❑❑ **What is a hydrocarbon?**

A hydrocarbon is a compound that contains both hydrogen and carbon.

❑❑ **Is a hydrocarbon hydrophilic or hydrophobic? Why?**

Hydrophobic. Remember that "like attracts like." Hydrocarbons are non-polar, whereas water is polar. Thus, hydrocarbons will not "attract" water or dissolve in water. Therefore, hydrocarbons are hydro*phobic,* which literally means "water-fearing".

❑❑ **What is the difference between a saturated and an unsaturated hydrocarbon?**

A *saturated* hydrocarbon is filled up with or "saturated" with hydrogens. Thus, no double bonds are found in saturated hydrocarbons. A hydrocarbon that is *unsaturated* does not have a full contingent of hydrogens. Therefore, an unsaturated hydrocarbon contains either a double or triple bond.

❑❑ **What is the group name for saturated hydrocarbons?**

Alkanes.

❑❑ **Would you classify alkanes as "highly reactive" or "relatively inert"?**

Alkanes are relatively inert. That is, they do not react with most substances.

❑❑ **What is the general "formula" for alkanes?**

General formula: C_nH_{2n+2}. An example of an alkane is CH_4 (methane). Alkanes form single bonds between carbon molecules.

❑❑ **What are two reactions that alkanes undergo?**

Combustion and halogenation.

❑❑ **What are the products of the following reaction? What is the name of this type of reaction?**

$$CH_4 + 2O_2 \rightarrow$$

This is a combustion reaction. A hydrocarbon is "burnt" with oxygen to form carbon dioxide, water, and heat energy. Thus, $CH_4 + 2O_2 \rightarrow CO_2 + H_2O$ + Energy.

❑❑ **What is the heat of combustion?**

The *heat of combustion* is the heat energy given off during the combustion reaction. The *higher the heat of combustion*, the *less stable* the carbon compound that was used in the reaction.

❑❑ **Which of the following will have a higher heat of combustion?**

$$CH_3\text{-}CH_2\text{-}CH_2\text{-}CH_3$$

$$\begin{array}{c} CH_3 \\ | \\ CH_3\text{-}CH_2\text{-}CH_3 \end{array}$$

The alkane on the right will have a higher heat of combustion. The branch on this alkane causes steric effects. Thus, the alkane on the right is less stable and therefore has a higher heat of combustion.

❑❑ **What is the product of the following reaction? By what mechanism does the reaction take place?**

$$R\text{-}H + Cl_2 \xrightarrow{light}$$

This is halogenation of an alkane. The reaction takes place by a *free radical* mechanism.

$$R\text{-}H + Cl_2 \xrightarrow{light} R\text{-}Cl + HCl$$

❑❑ **What is the catalyst in the free radical halogenation of an alkane?**

Light.

❑❑ **What is a free radical?**

A free radical is an element that has at least one unpaired electron.

❑❑ **Are free radicals very reactive or relatively inert?**

Free radicals are *very reactive* since they contain an unfilled outer electron shell.

❏❏ **What are the steps of the free radical reaction of R-H and Cl_2?**

Initiation: $Cl\text{-}Cl \xrightarrow{\text{light}} 2Cl\bullet$

Propagation: $R\text{-}H \; + \; Cl\bullet \longrightarrow R\bullet \; + \; HCl$

$R\bullet \; + \; Cl_2 \longrightarrow R\text{-}Cl \; + \; Cl\bullet$

Termination: $R\bullet \; + \; R\bullet \longrightarrow R\text{-}R$

$R\bullet \; + \; Cl\bullet \longrightarrow R\text{-}Cl$

$Cl\bullet \; + \; Cl\bullet \longrightarrow Cl\text{-}Cl$

❏❏ **What is the difference between a homolytic and a heterolytic process?**

In a homolytic process, symmetrical cleavage between two molecules takes place. In a heterolytic process, asymmetrical cleavage takes place.

$X \!\overset{\bullet}{\underset{\bullet}{}}\! Y \longrightarrow X^\bullet \; + \; Y^\bullet$ $\qquad\qquad$ $X \!\overset{\bullet}{\underset{\bullet}{}}\! Y \longrightarrow X^+ \; + \; \overset{\bullet}{\underset{\bullet}{}}Y^-$

Homolytic Bond Cleavage $\qquad\qquad$ Heterolytic Bond Cleavage

❏❏ **What are the three steps in the free radical halogenation of an alkane?**

1- Initiation (formation of halogen radical).
2- Propagation (formation of product and halogen radical).
3- Termination (formation of end products).

❏❏ **What is the stability order of free radicals?**

A tertiary (3°) radical is more stable than a secondary (2°) radical which is more stable than a primary (1°) radical.

❏❏ **Why do free radicals exhibit the order of reactivity that was noted in the previous question?**

The more substituted the alkyl radical (e.g., tertiary), the more the electrons are able to delocalize and distribute charge. Thus, the more substituted, the more stable.

❑❑ **Name the following molecules and place them in order from most stable to least stable.**

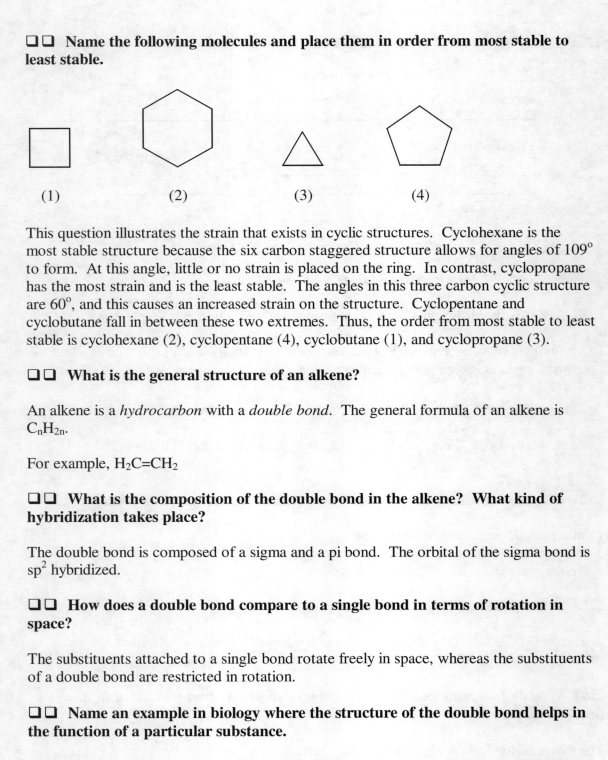

(1)   (2)   (3)   (4)

This question illustrates the strain that exists in cyclic structures. Cyclohexane is the most stable structure because the six carbon staggered structure allows for angles of 109° to form. At this angle, little or no strain is placed on the ring. In contrast, cyclopropane has the most strain and is the least stable. The angles in this three carbon cyclic structure are 60°, and this causes an increased strain on the structure. Cyclopentane and cyclobutane fall in between these two extremes. Thus, the order from most stable to least stable is cyclohexane (2), cyclopentane (4), cyclobutane (1), and cyclopropane (3).

❑❑ **What is the general structure of an alkene?**

An alkene is a *hydrocarbon* with a *double bond*. The general formula of an alkene is C_nH_{2n}.

For example, $H_2C=CH_2$

❑❑ **What is the composition of the double bond in the alkene? What kind of hybridization takes place?**

The double bond is composed of a sigma and a pi bond. The orbital of the sigma bond is sp^2 hybridized.

❑❑ **How does a double bond compare to a single bond in terms of rotation in space?**

The substituents attached to a single bond rotate freely in space, whereas the substituents of a double bond are restricted in rotation.

❑❑ **Name an example in biology where the structure of the double bond helps in the function of a particular substance.**

Peptide chains. The firm or rigid character of the double bond enables strings of amino acids to maintain a strong "backbone."

❑❑ **Label the following structures cis or trans. Explain.**

$$CH_3 \quad\quad CH_3$$
$$C = C$$
$$H \quad\quad H$$

$$H \quad\quad CH_3$$
$$C = C$$
$$CH_3 \quad\quad H$$

The structure on the left is the cis isomer of 2-butene, and the structure on the right is the trans isomer. Cis and trans isomers have the same structural formula but different spatial arrangement of atoms. If both of the methyl groups are on the *same* side of the double bond, this is the *cis* form. If both of the substituents are on *opposite* sides of the double bond, this is referred to as the *trans* form.

❑❑ **Label the following structures cis or trans. Explain your answer.**

$$CH_3 \quad\quad H$$
$$C = C$$
$$CH_3 \quad\quad H$$

$$H \quad\quad CH_3$$
$$C = C$$
$$H \quad\quad CH_3$$

This is a trick question as these two structures are identical. Remember, if both of the substituents attached to one of the carbons are identical, then cis and trans do not apply (i.e., the molecules are identical).

❑❑ **Label the following structures cis or trans. Explain your answer.**

$$CH_3 \quad\quad Cl$$
$$C = C$$
$$H \quad\quad H$$

$$CH_3 \quad\quad H$$
$$C = C$$
$$H \quad\quad Cl$$

This is also a trick question as cis and trans can only be used for naming disubstituted molecules. For molecules with three different substituents, a different naming system must be used. The system used is the E and Z nomenclature. In this example, the structure on the left is Z, and the structure on the right is E.

❑❑ **Which are more stable, cis or trans isomers? Why?**

Trans isomers are generally more stable than cis. The trans form allows substituents to spread apart and avoid steric hindrance. Thus, the trans form is more stable.

❑❑ **Is this an E or a Z configuration?**

$$\underset{\substack{\displaystyle \text{H}}}{\overset{\substack{\displaystyle \text{Cl}}}{\text{C}}} = \underset{\substack{\displaystyle \text{CH}_3}}{\overset{\substack{\displaystyle \text{Br}}}{\text{C}}}$$

This is an example of Z configuration. The method to determine this is as follows:

1- Compare the atomic number of the two substituents attached to the same carbon.
2- Label the substituent with the higher atomic number as "HIGH" and the substituent with the lower atomic number as "LOW."
3- Now compare the two substituents on the same side of the double bond as you would when determining cis or trans.
4- If the two substituents are the *same priority* (e.g., HIGH), then they are in Z configuration. If the two substituents are *not the same priority,* then they are in E configuration.

Memory Tip: *Zee Zame Zide*

High Cl   Br High

$$\text{C} = \text{C}$$

Low H   CH₃ Low

❑❑ **Is the following compound Z or E?**

$$\underset{\substack{\displaystyle \text{H}}}{\overset{\substack{\displaystyle \text{Cl}}}{\text{C}}} = \underset{\substack{\displaystyle \text{Br}}}{\overset{\substack{\displaystyle \text{H}}}{\text{C}}}$$

This compound is designated E because the two substituents on the same side of the double bond are not of the same priority. See below:

HIGH   Cl   H   LOW

$$\text{C} = \text{C}$$

LOW   H   Br   HIGH

❏❏ **Place the following bonds in order from longest to shortest:**

A) $CH_2=CH_2$ **B) H_3C-CH_3**   **C) $HC\equiv CH$**

B > A > C. *Increasing* the number of bonds *decreases the length* of the bonds. Thus, a single bond is longer than a double bond, which is longer than a triple bond.

❏❏ **As the length of the alkene increases, what happens to the boiling point? Why?**

Increases. The increase in the length of the alkene leads to an increase in the amount of intermolecular attractive forces. The increased intermolecular forces therefore cause a higher boiling point.

❏❏ **As the number of branches in an alkene increases, what happens to the boiling point? Why?**

Decreases. More branches cause increased steric hindrance. These branches "push" the molecules apart, making them more prone to boiling when heat is applied. Therefore, the boiling point is decreased.

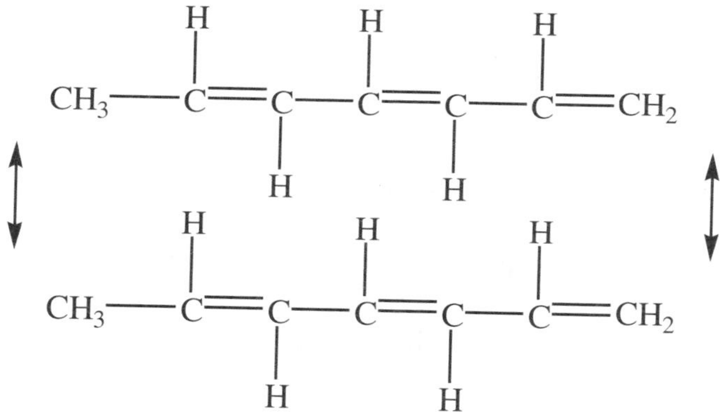

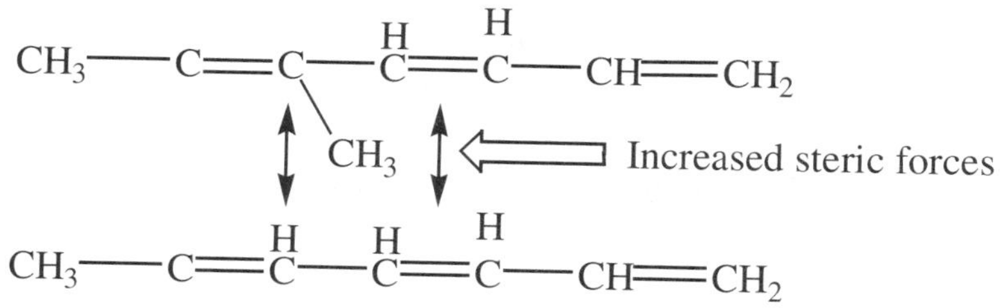

❏❏ **Which of the following alkenes is more stable?**

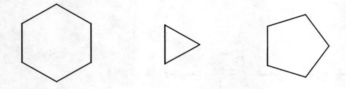

The alkene on the left is more stable. Remember that the *more carbons substituted* on the alkene, the *more stable* the alkene.

❏❏ **Which have more energy, single or double bonds?**

As the number of bonds increases, the energy of the bonds also increases. Thus, a triple bond has more energy than a double bond, which has more energy than a single bond.

❏❏ **Label the following cyclic hydrocarbons:**

Cyclohexane, cyclopropane, and cyclopentane.

❏❏ **Which has a higher boiling point…cyclohexane or hexane?**

Cyclohexane. Cyclic alkanes tend to have higher boiling points than their noncyclic counterparts.

❏❏ **Alkanes are most soluble in which of the following: water, ether, ethanol, or sodium chloride?**

Alkanes are most soluble in ether because it is non-polar. All of the other choices (i.e. , water, ethanol, and sodium chloride) are polar. Like dissolves like.

❏❏ **What are the three general categories of reactions that an alkene can undergo?**

1. Electrophilic addition.
2. Reduction.
3. Oxidation.

❏❏ **What is an electrophile?**

Electrophile literally means "electron-loving." These substances are electron poor and would love to gain or accept electrons.

❏❏ **What is the mechanism of electrophilic addition to an alkene?**

An electrophile is attacked by the double bond (i.e., the electrons) of the alkene. A number of reactions occur by this mechanism. Example:

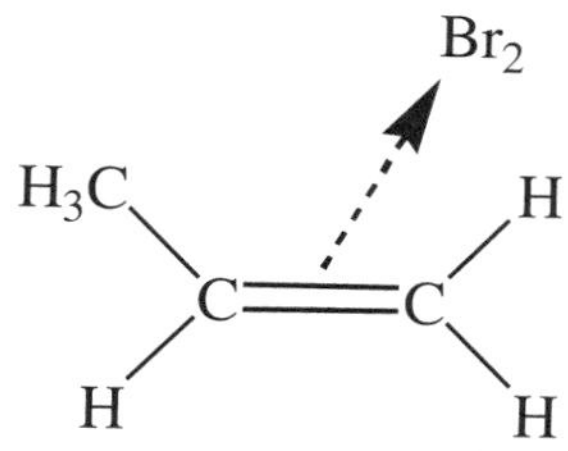

❏❏ **What is the product of the following reaction? What is the mechanism of the reaction?**

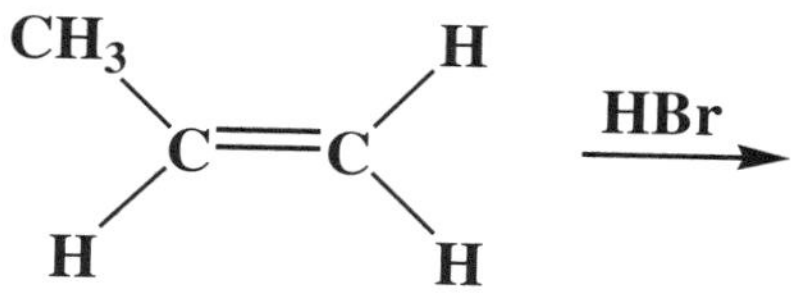

This is an electrophilic addition reaction. The reaction takes place by carbocation intermediate. As noted below, the electrons of the double bond attack H-Br (i.e., the electrophile). The electrons from the double bond form a bond with the hydrogen and a carbocation is formed on the adjacent carbon. In turn, the electron from hydrogen is transferred to the bromine, forming Br⁻. The negatively charged bromine is attracted to the positively charged carbocation. This mechanism is similar to many of the other alkene addition reactions.

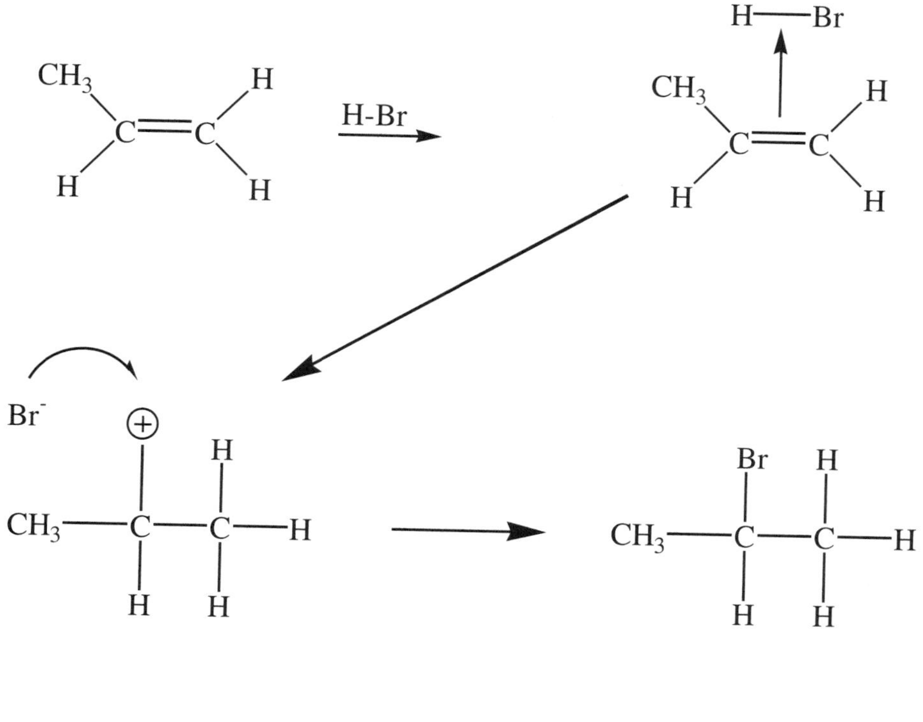

❑❑ **What is a carbocation?**

A carbocation is a carbon molecule with a positive charge.

❑❑ **What are the correct products of the following reaction? How do you determine this?**

The correct products of the reaction are A. A previous question revealed that this reaction takes place via a carbocation mechanism. Remember that *the carbocation always forms on the more substituted (i.e., more stable) carbon.* Thus, the hydrogen from the HBr binds to the less substituted side, and a carbocation forms on the more substituted side. The negatively charged Br then attaches to the carbocation site. The concept that the carbocation forms on the most substituted carbon is *Markovnikov's rule.*

❑❑ **Who is Markovnikov (for interest only)? Restate his rule.**

Vladimir Markovnikov was a Russian chemist who proposed in 1869 what later became Markovnikov's rule: In the addition of HX to an alkene, the acid hydrogen becomes attached to the carbon with fewer alkyl substituents, and the X group becomes attached to the carbon with more alkyl substituents.

❑❑ **What are the products of the following reaction? Does this follow Markovnikov's rule or not?**

This reaction does not follow Markovnikov's rule. This reaction takes place by free radical addition rather than by carbocation. The addition of peroxide (H_2O_2) is responsible for the change in mechanism. This reaction is considered *Anti-Markovnikov.*

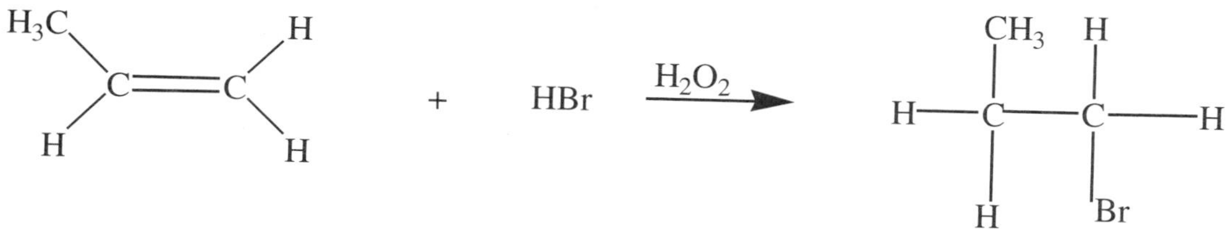

❑❑ **What are the products of the following reaction? What stereochemistry will the products exhibit?**

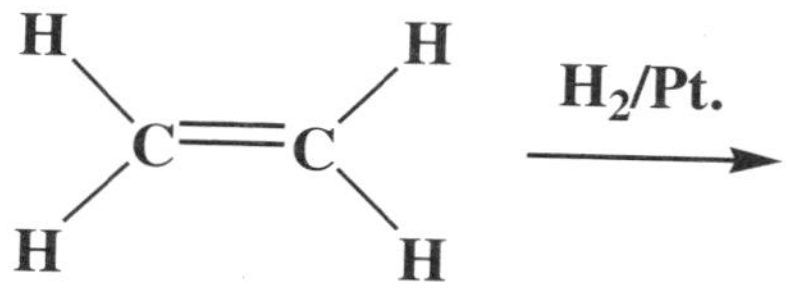

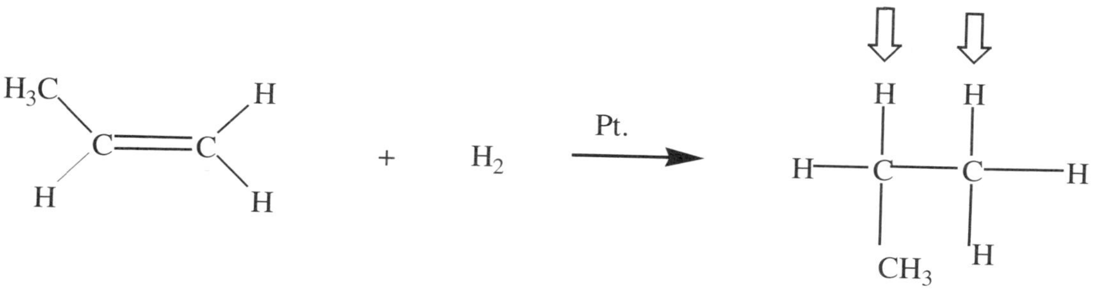

This is an example of hydrogenation of an alkene. The products are an alkane as noted. The stereochemistry of this reaction is *syn*. That means that both hydrogens are on the same side. This is in contrast to *anti* stereochemistry which means that the substituents would be added to opposite sides. If the molecule can add to either side without regard to syn or anti, the stereochemistry is termed *random*.

❑❑ **Which of the following will have a higher heat of hydrogenation?**

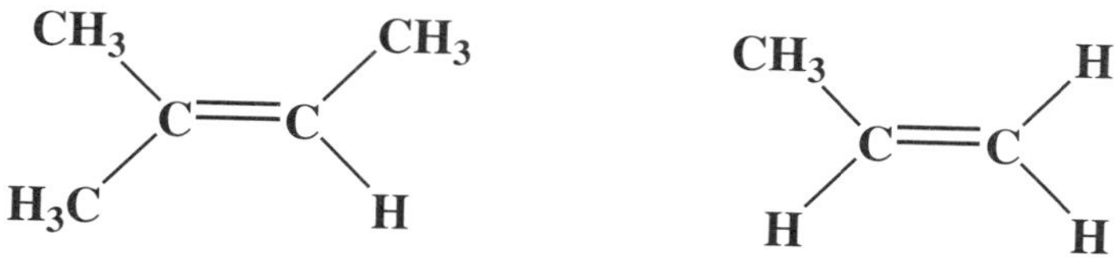

The compound on the right will have a higher heat of hydrogenation. The heat of hydrogenation is the amount of heat given off during hydrogenation of an alkene (previous reaction). The less stable (less substituted) carbon will have a higher heat of hydrogenation than a more stable (more substituted) carbon.

❏❏ **Fill in the products for the following electrophilic addition reactions. Note the regiochemistry (Markovnikov or Anti-Mark) and the stereochemistry (syn, anti, or random) of the reactions.**

1)

H_3C ⟍   ⟋ H
        $C = C$
H ⟋   ⟍ H + Br_2 ⟶

2)

H_3C ⟍   ⟋ H
        $C = C$
H ⟋   ⟍ H +   HBr   ⟶

3)

H_3C ⟍   ⟋ H
        $C = C$ H_2O_2
H ⟋   ⟍ H +   HBr   ⟶

4)

H_3C ⟍   ⟋ H
        $C = C$ Pt.
H ⟋   ⟍ H + H_2 ⟶

1)

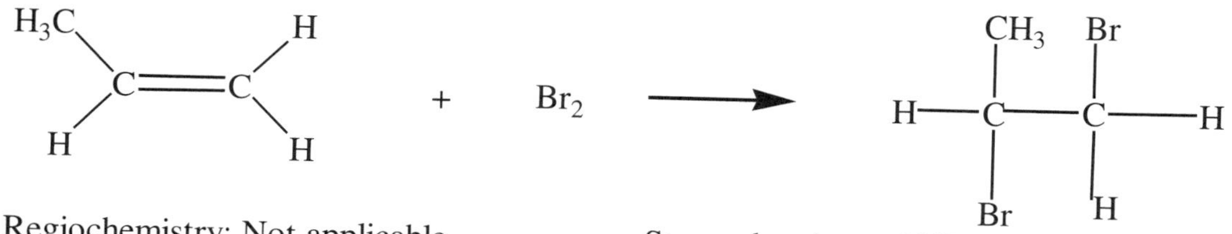

H_3C H
   C = C
  H   H

+ Br_2 →

CH$_3$ Br
H—C——C—H
    Br   H

Regiochemistry: Not applicable

Stereochemistry: ANTI

2)

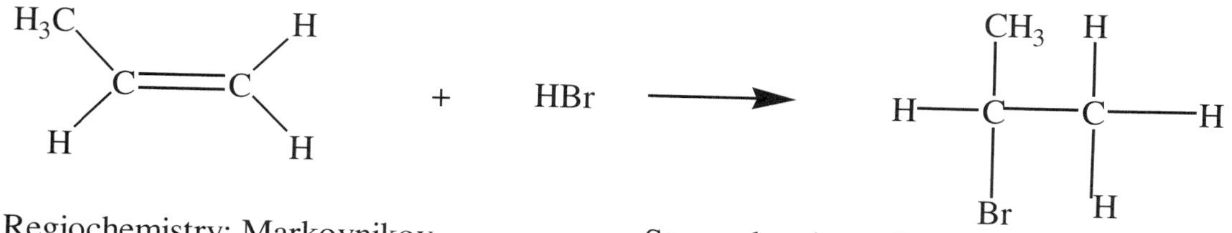

H_3C H
   C = C
  H   H

+   HBr   →

CH$_3$ H
H—C——C—H
    Br   H

Regiochemistry: Markovnikov

Stereochemistry: Random

3)

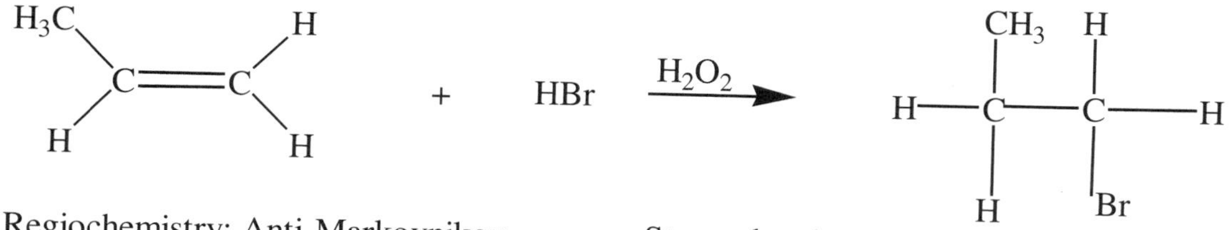

H_3C H
   C = C
  H   H

+   HBr $\xrightarrow{H_2O_2}$

CH$_3$ H
H—C——C—H
    H   Br

Regiochemistry: Anti-Markovnikov

Stereochemistry: Random

4)

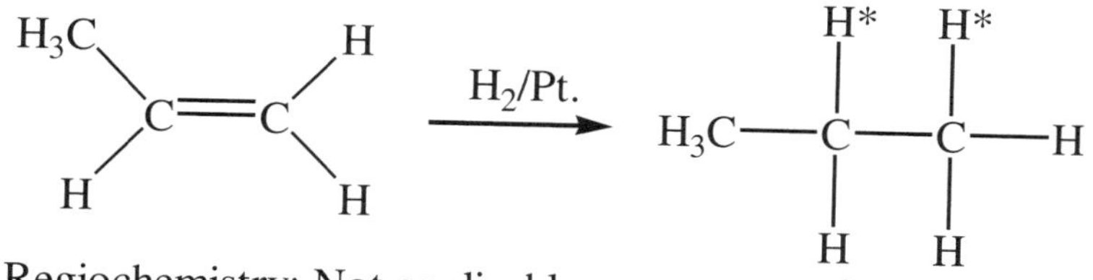

H_3C H
   C = C
  H   H

$\xrightarrow{H_2/Pt.}$

H*   H*
H_3C—C——C—H
     H   H

Regiochemistry: Not applicable

Stereochemistry: SYN

❑ ❑ What are the products of the following reaction?

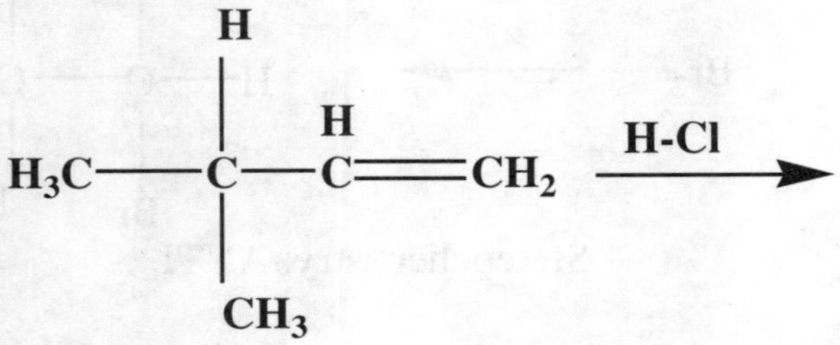

$$H_3C - \underset{\underset{CH_3}{|}}{\overset{\overset{H}{|}}{C}} - \overset{\overset{H}{|}}{C} = CH_2 \xrightarrow{\text{H-Cl}}$$

This is an example of a rearrangement. In this reaction, the hydrogen shifts position to allow the carbocation to form on the most substituted carbon. The same type of rearrangement may occur with a methyl group.

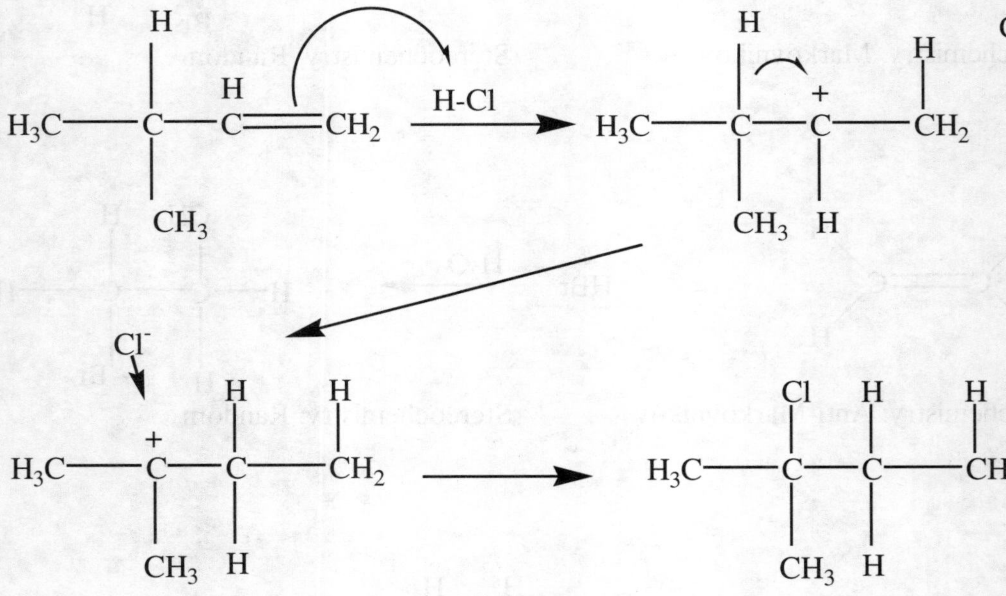

$$H_3C - \underset{\underset{CH_3}{|}}{\overset{\overset{H}{|}}{C}} - \overset{\overset{H}{|}}{C} = CH_2 \xrightarrow{\text{H-Cl}} H_3C - \underset{\underset{CH_3}{|}}{\overset{\overset{H}{|}}{C}} - \overset{\overset{+}{|}}{\underset{H}{C}} - CH_2 \quad Cl^-$$

$$H_3C - \overset{+}{\underset{\underset{CH_3}{|}}{C}} - \underset{\underset{H}{|}}{\overset{\overset{H}{|}}{C}} - CH_2 \xrightarrow{} H_3C - \underset{\underset{CH_3}{|}}{\overset{\overset{Cl}{|}}{C}} - \underset{\underset{H}{|}}{\overset{\overset{H}{|}}{C}} - \overset{\overset{H}{|}}{CH_2}$$

NOMENCLATURE

❑❑ **How are the "prefix" and the "suffix" in organic chemistry nomenclature determined?**

Prefix: Determined by the number of carbons in the carbon chain.
Suffix: Derived after determining the functional group involved. If more than one functional group is noted, the "highest priority" group should be determined.

❑❑ **What are the correct prefixes for the first ten carbon chains?**

PREFIX	# OF CARBONS
METH-	1
ETH-	2
PROP-	3
BUT-	4
PENT-	5
HEX-	6
HEPT-	7
OCT-	8
NON-	9
DEC-	10

❑❑ **What are the correct suffixes for the following functional groups:**

1- Aldehyde
2- Carboxylic acid
3- Alcohol
4- Ketone
5- Alkene
6- Alkane
7- Alkyne

1) –al 2) –oic or –oate 3) –ol 4) –one 5) –ene 6) –ane 7) –yne

❑❑ **How do you name a suffix of a molecule that has two functional groups present?**

Use the suffix of the molecule with the highest priority.

❑❑ **What is the order of priorities used for naming the suffixes of the following functional groups:**

Alkenes (-ene), Carboxylic acids (-oate), Amines (-amine), Aldehydes (-al), Alkynes (-yne), Ketones (-one), Alcohols (-ol), Alkanes (-ane)

Suffixes (from highest to lowest priority):
   Carboxylic acids (-oate) and derivatives
   Aldehydes (-al)
   Ketones (-one)
   Alcohols (-ol)
   Amines (-amine)
   Alkynes (-yne)
   Alkenes (-ene)
   Alkanes (-ane)

❑❑ **Label the following structures:**

Aldehyde   Alcohol   Ether   Ester
Ketone   Amine   Amide   Alkyl halide
Carboxylic Acid

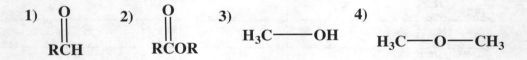

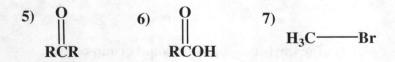

1) aldehyde, 2) ester, 3) alcohol, 4) ether, 5) ketone, 6) carboxylic acid, 7) alkyl halide

❑❑ What are the general rules for nomenclature?

General rules for nomenclature (abbreviated and to the point):
1. Find the LONGEST CHAIN → NAME IT.
   Prefix: Number of carbons in chain determines (as noted above).
   Suffix: Derived after determining the functional group involved. If more than one functional group is noted, the "highest priority" group should be determined.
2. Number the chain, starting from end closest to functional group.
3. Identify any substituents and their locations (1-methyl, 2-methyl, etc.)
4. If there is more than one of the same substituent, then use di- (two), tri- (three), tetra- (four), etc.
5. List alphabetically without regard to di, tri, tetra, etc.

❑❑ Name the following compound according to IUPAC nomenclature:

$$CH_3$$
$$|$$
$$CH_3CClCH_2CH_2CH_2CH_3$$

2-chloro-2-methylhexane.

❑❑ Name the following compound according to IUPAC nomenclature:

$$CH_3$$
$$|$$
$$CH_3CHCClHCH_2CH_2CH_3$$

3-chloro-2-methylhexane.

❑❑ Name the following compound according to IUPAC nomenclature:

$$O$$
$$||$$
$$CH_3CH_2CH$$

Propanal.

❑❑ Name the following compound according to IUPAC nomenclature:

$$CH_3CH_2CH_2CH_3$$
$$\backslash$$
$$CH_2CH_2CH_3$$

3-methylhexane. Remember to count the longest chain! If you did not, you are likely trying to figure out why this is named as a hexane instead of a butane.

CARBON BONDING

❑❑ **How many electrons does carbon have in its outer shell?**

Carbon has 4 electrons in the outer shell.

❑❑ **In what orbitals are the electrons in carbon's outer shell found?**

S orbital: 2 electrons
Px: 1 electron
Py: 1 electron
Pz: 0 electron

❑❑ **How do the electrons in carbon's outer shell rearrange when excited? Why is this important?**

One of the two electrons in the S orbital jumps to the Pz orbital. Thus,

S orbital: 1 electron
Px: 1 electron
Py: 1 electron
Pz: 1 electron

This is important in that each of these four orbitals then participates in the hybridization of the carbon molecule. That is, the S orbital hybridizes with one or more of the P orbitals.

❑❑ **What is an sp³ hybridized carbon?**

This is a hybrid of the four orbitals previously mentioned. Note how the S orbital combines with three P orbitals. Hence the term sp^3.

❑❑ **What is an sp² carbon?**

This is a hybrid of the S orbital and two P orbitals. Hence the term sp^2. The remaining P orbital forms a pi bond.

❑❑ **What is an sp^1 carbon?**

This is a hybrid of the S orbital and one P orbital. Hence the term sp^1. The remaining two P orbitals each form a pi bond.

$$H-C\equiv C-H$$

NUCLEOPHILIC SUBSTITUTION REACTIONS

❑❑ **What are the two types of nucleophilic substitution reactions called?**

S_N1 and S_N2.

❑❑ **What do "S_N1" and "S_N2" stand for?**

S = substitution   1 = unimolecular (first-order reaction)
N = nucleophilic   2 = bimolecular (second-order reaction)

❑❑ **What is a nucleophile?**

Nucleophile literally means "nucleus-loving." These are substances that are electron rich and would love to "attack" a nucleus which is electron deficient.

❑❑ **What is an electrophile?**

Electrophile literally means "electron-loving." These substances are electron poor and would love to gain or accept electrons.

❑❑ **What is the intermediate in the S_N1 reaction?**

S_N1 reactions work via a *CARBOCATION* intermediate.

❑❑ **How does a carbocation form in the S_N1 reaction?**

A substrate (which is an electrophile) forms a carbocation when a LEAVING GROUP breaks off or "leaves" the substrate. When the leaving group takes off (and with it electrons), a positive charge remains on the substrate. This is the carbocation. Below is an example of an S_N1 reaction. Note that –OH receives a hydrogen from HBr which makes it into a good leaving group.

❏❏ **Label the following carbons as either primary, secondary, or tertiary carbons:**

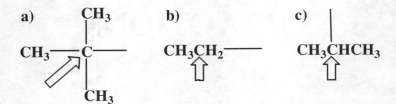

a) Tertiary
b) Primary
c) Secondary

Primary, secondary, and tertiary carbon refers to the number of carbon atoms that are directly attached to the carbon in question. A primary carbon is attached to only one carbon; the secondary to two; the tertiary to three.

❏❏ **When a carbocation forms, it may be on a primary, secondary, or tertiary substituted carbon. Which of these form the most stable carbocation?**

Tertiary (most stable) > Secondary > Primary.

❏❏ **What is the rate-limiting step of an S_N1 reaction?**

The rate-limiting step of an S_N1 reaction is the formation of the carbocation intermediate. The rate of the S_N1 reaction is thus ONLY dependent upon the *SUBSTRATE* which forms the carbocation. The nucleophile has NO effect on the rate of the reaction. Hence, S_N**1** – **FIRST**-ORDER reaction rate.

❏❏ **What are the products of an S_N1 reaction when the substrate is a pure enantiomer?**

Racemic products.

❏❏ **What are "racemic" products?**

Racemic products consist of 50% of one enantiomer and 50% of the other (i.e., 50% R and 50% S). They are formed because a carbocation is equally likely to be attacked from the front as it is the back.

❏❏ **Are racemic products optically active?**

No. Racemic products contain 50% R and 50% S configuration. This 50:50 ratio balances out each other's tendency to rotate in plane polarized light. Thus, no rotation is observed.

❑❑ **What does "S$_N$2" stand for?**

S = substitution
$_N$ = nucleophilic
2 = bimolecular

❑❑ **What is the reactivity order of an S$_N$2 reaction? Why?**

Primary (1°) > Secondary (2°) > Tertiary (3°)
An S$_N$2 reaction is more favorable with less steric hindrance. The fewer substituents on the carbon, the more favorable the reaction.

❑❑ **What is the mechanism of an S$_N$2 reaction? Is a carbocation involved?**

No, a carbocation is not involved. An S$_N$2 reaction occurs when a nucleophile attacks a substrate from the "backside." The backside attack occurs as noted in the example below.

Backside attack

$$H_3C-\underset{\underset{H}{|}}{\overset{\overset{H}{|}}{C}}-OH \quad \xrightarrow{HBr} \quad H_3C-\underset{\underset{H}{|}}{\overset{\overset{H}{|}}{C}}-\overset{+}{O}H \quad \longrightarrow \quad H_3C-\underset{\underset{H}{|}}{\overset{\overset{H}{|}}{C}}-Br$$

Leaving group

❑❑ **What happens to the products of an S$_N$2 reaction if the substrate is a chiral carbon?**

Inversion of configuration of the products.

❑❑ **What are the *general* characteristics of a good nucleophile?**

A good nucleophile follows some general trends:
1. Usually *increases going down column* in periodic table
   Example: HS- is better nucleophile than HO-.
2. Nucleophilicity roughly parallels basicity: the *more basic* → *the better nucleophile.*

❑❑ **What kinds of nucleophiles are best for an S$_N$1 reaction?**

Non-basic nucleophiles such as CH_3CH_2OH are best for S$_N$1 reactions.

❑❑ **What is the *general* criterion for a good leaving group?**

In general, *weaker bases* make *better* leaving groups.

❏❏ **What is the reactivity order of the following leaving groups?**

I-, Br-, H_2O, Cl-, Tosylate

Decreasing reactivity: Tosylate- > I- > Br- > Cl- ≅ H_2O.

❏❏ **Is ⁻OH a good or a bad leaving group?**

-OH is a BAD leaving group. If -OH is protonated by an acid and becomes H_2O, then it is a GOOD leaving group. BUT remember that -OH *must* receive a H^+ first!

❏❏ **What are the products of the following reaction?**

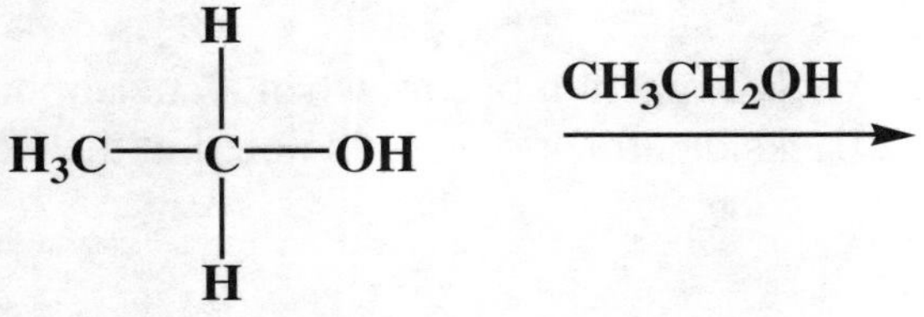

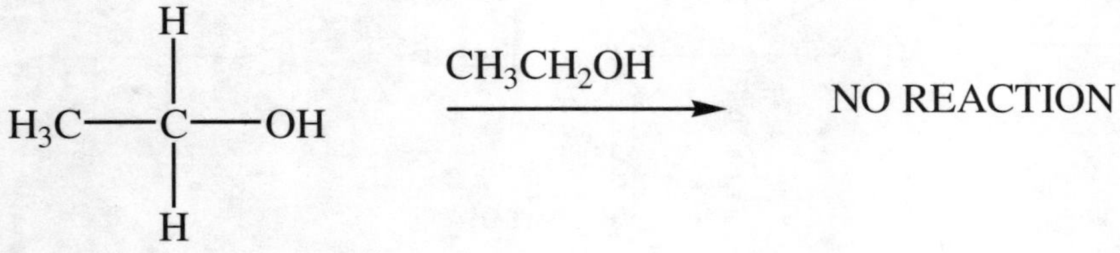

As noted in the previous question, -OH is a bad leaving group unless it is protonated. Thus, this equation will result in no reaction.

❏❏ **What type of solvent is best for S_N2 reactions?**

Polar, aprotic solvents.

❏❏ **What type of solvent is best for S_N1 reactions?**

Polar, protic solvents.

❏❏ **How do you determine if a reaction is S_N1, S_N2, E1, E2?**

This is not a simple answer. The following method may help in determining the nature of the reaction.

1. Find the leaving group in the chemical reaction.
2. Identify the carbon (tertiary, secondary, primary) that the leaving group is attached to.

Primary carbon: Either an S_N1 or an E2 reaction
E2 → only if very strong base such as tert-butoxide
S_N2 → with good nucleophile

Secondary carbon: Any of the four (S_N1, E1, S_N2, E2)
-Any of the reactions may take place on a secondary carbon. In this case, look at the characteristics of each type of reaction.

Tertiary carbon: Either S_N1, E1, or E2
S_N1 → with non-basic nucleophile
E2 → with base
E1 → typically occurs with S_N1 reaction.

❑❑ **Are the following reactions S_N1 or S_N2?**
a)

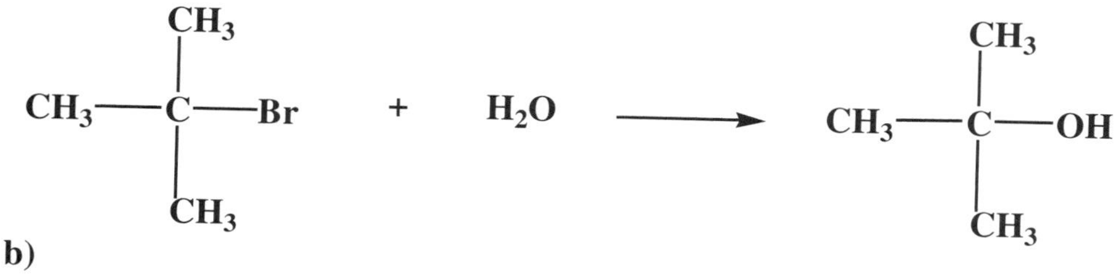

$$CH_3-\underset{\underset{CH_3}{|}}{\overset{\overset{CH_3}{|}}{C}}-Br \quad + \quad H_2O \quad \longrightarrow \quad CH_3-\underset{\underset{CH_3}{|}}{\overset{\overset{CH_3}{|}}{C}}-OH$$

b)
CH_3Br + CN^- → CH_3CN + Br^-

Reaction "a" is an example of an S_N1 reaction. Note that the bromide is attached to a tertiary carbon. Reaction "b" is an example of an S_N2 reaction.

❑❑ **Label the following chart:**

	S_N1	S_N2
Reaction order		
Mechanism		
Reactivity		
Products (if chiral)		
Rearrangements?		
Favorable solvent		

	S_N1	S_N2
Reaction order	First-order reaction Rate=k [substrate]	Second-order reaction Rate=k [substrate] [Nu]
Mechanism	Carbocation	Backside attack
Reactivity	$3° > 2° > 1°$	$1° > 2°$
Products (if chiral)	Racemic	Inverted configuration
Rearrangements?	Yes (because of carbocation)	No
Favorable solvent	Polar protic	Polar aprotic

ALDEHYDES AND KETONES

❑❑   **What is the general formula for an aldehyde? What is the general formula for a ketone?**

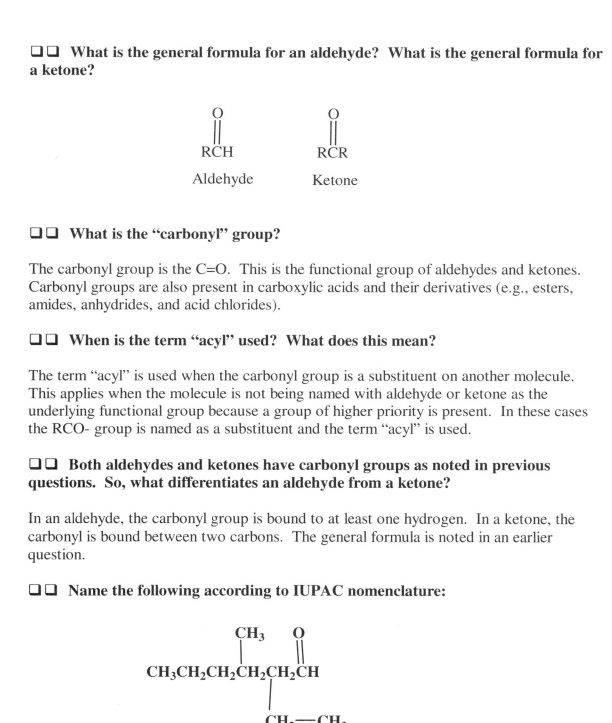

❑❑   **What is the "carbonyl" group?**

The carbonyl group is the C=O. This is the functional group of aldehydes and ketones. Carbonyl groups are also present in carboxylic acids and their derivatives (e.g., esters, amides, anhydrides, and acid chlorides).

❑❑   **When is the term "acyl" used? What does this mean?**

The term "acyl" is used when the carbonyl group is a substituent on another molecule. This applies when the molecule is not being named with aldehyde or ketone as the underlying functional group because a group of higher priority is present. In these cases the RCO- group is named as a substituent and the term "acyl" is used.

❑❑   **Both aldehydes and ketones have carbonyl groups as noted in previous questions. So, what differentiates an aldehyde from a ketone?**

In an aldehyde, the carbonyl group is bound to at least one hydrogen. In a ketone, the carbonyl is bound between two carbons. The general formula is noted in an earlier question.

❑❑   **Name the following according to IUPAC nomenclature:**

2-ethyl-3-methyl-hexanal. This is determined as follows:

Find the longest chain that *contains the aldehyde.**

Number the chain starting with the carbonyl carbon.

Name the prefix according to the standard rules (see nomenclature section).

Name the suffix: -al for aldehyde.

Label and name substituents as described for general nomenclature.

*Remember to choose the longest chain that contains the aldehyde. If the longest chain were chosen *excluding the aldehyde*, then the above example would have been named as a seven carbon chain.

❑❑ **Name the following:**

$$\overset{\displaystyle O}{\overset{\displaystyle \|}{CH_3CH_2CCH_3}}$$

2-butanone. Ketones are named in a similar fashion to aldehydes (see previous question). Numbering of the ketone begins at the end of the chain closest to the carbonyl group. Also, the suffix –one is used instead of –al.

❑❑ **What is the distribution of charge on the carbonyl? How does this affect reactions which take place here?**

The electronegativity of the oxygen molecule creates a partial negative charge on the oxygen and a partial positive charge on the carbon. Take a moment to understand and memorize this fact. Understanding this is key to understanding the chemistry/reactions of aldehydes, ketones, and carboxylic acids.

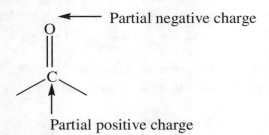

❑❑ **Place the following in order from lowest to highest boiling point:**

$$CH_3CH_2CH_2CH_2\text{-}OH \qquad \overset{\displaystyle O}{\overset{\displaystyle \|}{CH_3CH_2CCH_3}} \qquad CH_3CH_2CH_2CH_3$$

1   2   3

3 (lowest), 2, 1 (highest). Aldehydes and ketones are polar molecules and will have higher boiling points than their hydrocarbon counterparts. Alcohols are also polar and will form hydrogen bonds. Thus, alcohols have higher boiling points than their aldehyde, ketone, or hydrocarbon counterparts.

❑❑ **Which react faster, aldehydes or ketones? Why?**

Aldehydes react faster than ketones. The additional carbon group of the ketone serves to stabilize it. The aldehyde is less stable and therefore more reactive.

❑❑ **List some of the ways that aldehydes/ketones are formed.**

1. Oxidation of alcohols
2. Friedel-Crafts acylation (ketones only)
3. Ozonolysis of alkenes

❑❑ **What are the major reactions that aldehydes and ketones undergo?**

1. Oxidation
2. Addition (nucleophilic)
3. Hydration
4. Cyanohydrin
5. Hydride reduction
6. Formation of acetal/ketal/hemiacetal/hemiketal
7. Imine/enamine formation (addition, then elimination)
8. Grignard reagents
9. Aldol condensation

❑❑ **What is the product of the following reaction? What type of reaction is this?**

$$
\underset{CH_3CH}{\overset{O}{\|}} \quad \xrightarrow[\text{NH}_4\text{OH, H}_2\text{O}]{\text{Ag}_2\text{O}}
$$

$$
\underset{CH_3CH}{\overset{O}{\|}} \quad \xrightarrow[\text{NH}_4\text{OH, H}_2\text{O}]{\text{Ag}_2\text{O}} \quad \underset{CH_3COH}{\overset{O}{\|}}
$$

This is an example of an oxidation reaction. The oxidation agent in this reaction is the Tollens reagent. The difference between this reagent and others such as the Jones reagent is probably not important for the MCAT, but the Tollens reagent does not disrupt other functional groups including the carbon-carbon double bond. Also, the Tollens reagent turns the walls of the flask silver when reacting. The metallic silver indicates that an aldehyde is present.

Safety tip: *Oxidation* (i.e., losing electrons) can be quickly identified in organic reactions as *either gaining of oxygen or losing hydrogen*. Note the gain of oxygen in the above reaction. Also note that oxidizing agents typically have a number of oxygen molecules.

❑❑ **What are the products of the following reaction? What general category does this reaction fall under? What specific type of reaction is this?**

$$CH_3\overset{\displaystyle O}{\overset{\|}{C}}H \xrightarrow{\text{HCN}}$$

$$CH_3\overset{\displaystyle O}{\overset{\|}{C}}H \xrightarrow{\text{HCN}} CH_3\overset{\displaystyle OH}{\underset{\displaystyle H}{\overset{|}{\underset{|}{C}}}}{-}CN$$

This is an addition reaction, specifically a cyanohydrin addition. The key to understanding this reaction is understanding the chemistry of the carbonyl group. Remember that oxygen has a partial negative charge and carbon has a partial positive charge. This charge polarity is created by the electronegativity of the oxygen. The partial positive charge on the carbon is a perfect "target" for any negative charge, in this case -CN. Thus, the carbon is an electrophile (i.e., electron-loving) and the group attaching is a nucleophile (i.e., nucleus-loving). In this case, the negative -CN attaches to the partial positive carbon. In addition, the hydrogen from the HCN protonates the oxygen, which has three lone pairs of electrons. Thus, an –OH is formed. Understanding this mechanism will help through all of the addition reactions of aldehydes and ketones.

❑❑ **What are the products of the following reaction?**

$$CH_3\overset{\displaystyle O}{\overset{\|}{C}}H \xrightarrow{\text{NaBH}_4}$$

$$CH_3\overset{\displaystyle O}{\overset{\|}{C}}H \xrightarrow{\text{NaBH}_4} CH_3CH_2\overset{\displaystyle OH}{\overset{|}{}}$$

This is another example of an addition reaction. In this case, hydrogen is added to the aldehyde and the reaction is a *reduction* (gains electrons). Again, the key to understanding this reaction is understanding the chemistry of the carbonyl group. Remember that oxygen has a partial negative charge and carbon has a partial positive charge. This charge polarity is created by the electronegativity of the oxygen. The partial positive charge on the carbon is a perfect "target" for any negative charge. Thus, the carbon is an electrophile (i.e., electron-loving) and the group attaching is a nucleophile (i.e., nucleus-loving). In this particular reaction, the negative hydrogen from $NaBH_4$ attacks the partial positive carbon. In addition, a hydrogen from the acid (H_3O^+) protonates the oxygen, which contains three lone pair electrons. Note that this reaction is a *reduction* reaction. The *addition of hydrogen* can be used to quickly identify the reaction as a reduction reaction.

❏❏ **What are the products of the following reaction? What type of reaction is this?**

This is a hemiacetal/acetal reaction, and the products are as follows:

❏❏ **In chemistry experiments, what role does the acetal group play?**

The acetal serves as a good "protecting group." That is, since the acetal is inert to most substances, this "protects" the molecules in question from undergoing unwanted reactions. An acetal reaction can be reversed with acid.

❏❏ **What biological molecule undergoes the hemiacetal/acetal reaction?**

Carbohydrates undergo this reaction as they are transformed from straight chains to ring formation. This results in the formation of hemiacetals. Further reaction with –OR group sometimes occurs, forming acetals. See carbohydrate section for more information.

❏❏   **What is the product of the following reaction?**

$$\underset{\underset{\displaystyle |}{\overset{\displaystyle OCH_3}{\overset{|}{C}}}}{} \quad OCH_2CH_3 \qquad \xrightarrow[\displaystyle H_2O]{\displaystyle H_3O+}$$

Though acetals are inert to most substances, they do react with acid. Deriving the products may not be easy, but the following method may help.

Trick for deriving products for reverse (breakdown of) acetal reaction:

1. Find the point of attachment (the carbon that the two oxygens attach to).
2. Eliminate the bond between the oxygen molecules and the carbon.
3. Add hydrogen to the oxygen molecules.
4. Add a double bonded oxygen to the "point of attachment" carbon.

❏❏   **What are the products of the following reaction? What type of reaction is this?**

$$\underset{CH_3CH}{\overset{\displaystyle \overset{O}{\|}}{}} \quad + \quad \underset{CH_3CH}{\overset{\displaystyle \overset{O}{\|}}{}}$$

This is an example of an aldol condensation reaction. The products are displayed below.

Acid or Base Catalyst   May undergo further dehydration
                                                     depending on reaction conditions

❏❏   **T/F: Aldehydes react faster than ketones.**

True.

❑❑   **T/F: Aldehydes are more stable than ketones.**

False.

❑❑   **T/F: An aldehyde has a higher boiling point than an equivalent size hydrocarbon.**

True.

❑❑   **T/F: An aldehyde has a higher boiling point than an equivalent size alcohol.**

False.

ETHERS

❑❑ **What is the general formula for an ether?**

R-O-R

❑❑ **What is the product of the following reaction?**

$$CH_3\text{-}O\text{-}CH_2\text{-}CH_3 + MgBrCH_2CH_3 \rightarrow$$

No reaction occurs. Ethers are inert when reacted with Grignard reagents.

❑❑ **Are ethers considered "highly reactive" or "relatively inert"?**

Ethers are inert with most substances including Grignard reagents, nucleophiles, mild acids, bases, and halogens.

❑❑ **What is the product of the following reaction?**

$$CH_3\text{-}CH_2\text{-}O\text{-}CH_2\text{-}CH_3 + HBr \rightarrow$$

Though most substances are inert with ethers, acids will cleave ethers as shown here. $CH_3\text{-}CH_2\text{-}O\text{-}CH_2\text{-}CH_3 + HBr \rightarrow CH_3\text{-}CH_2\text{-}OH + CH_3\text{-}CH_2\text{-}Br$

❑❑ **What is the mechanism of the reaction between an acid and an ether?**

The reaction mechanism is typically S_N2. If a secondary or tertiary carbon is involved, the reaction can proceed by an S_N1 mechanism.

❑❑ **What is the hybridization of the oxygen orbital in an ether?**

The oxygen orbital is sp^3 hybridized.

❑❑ **Do ethers act as weak acids or weak bases?**

Ethers act as weak bases.

❑❑ **What is the name of the structure below? Is it considered an ether?**

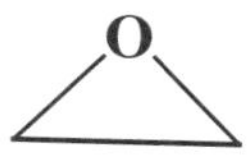

This is an epoxide. Yes.

❑❑ **What are the products of the following reaction?**

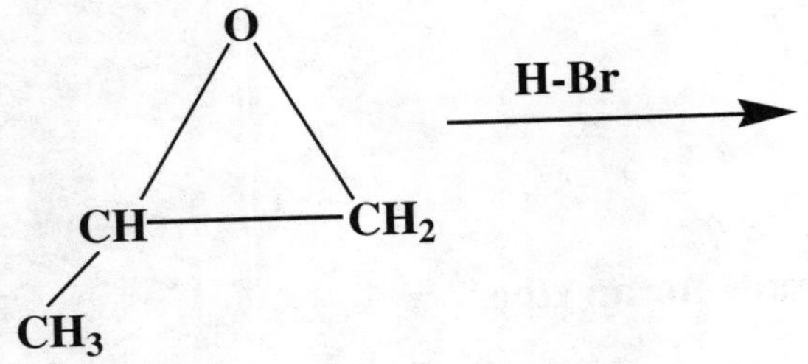

$$
\underset{\underset{CH_3}{|}}{CH}\overset{\displaystyle O}{\diagup\diagdown}CH_2 \quad \xrightarrow{\text{ H-Br }}
$$

This is an example of an epoxide reacting with an acid. The results are shown below.

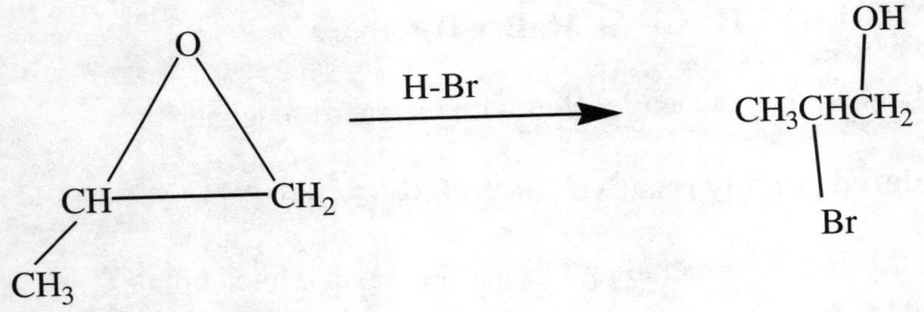

$$
\underset{\underset{CH_3}{|}}{CH}\overset{\displaystyle O}{\diagup\diagdown}CH_2 \quad \xrightarrow{\text{ H-Br }} \quad \underset{\underset{Br}{|}}{CH_3CHCH_2}\overset{OH}{}
$$

LIPIDS

❑❑ What is the definition of a lipid?

Lipids are compounds that are insoluble in aqueous solution, but soluble/extractable in organic (i.e., non-polar) solvents.

❑❑ What are some types of lipids?

Types of lipids include fats, oils, and cholesterol.

❑❑ What is saponification?

Saponification is hydrolysis of an ester with aqueous sodium hydroxide, yielding carboxylate salts and alcohols. See below. This reaction is important, as saponification is used to produce soaps from fats.

❑❑ What is a phospholipid?

A phospholipid is an ester of phosphoric acid H_3PO_4. A phospholipid contains both a non-polar tail and a charged head.

❑❑ How does the structure of a phospholipid play a role in its function in the cell membrane?

The nature of the phospholipid allows for a bilayer to form the cell membrane. The hydrophobic tails face and form the inside of the cell membrane, and the charged heads face and form the exterior of the cell membrane.

❑❑ Where in the digestive tract are lipids broken down?

Small intestine.

❏❏   **What substance facilitates the digestion of lipids? Where is this substance produced and stored?**

Bile. Bile is formed in the liver and stored in the gallbladder. Bile is delivered to the small intestine via ducts. In the small intestine, bile emulsifies fats and facilitates breakdown of the lipid.

❏❏   **After lipids are broken down in the digestive tract, what structure picks up the remains?**

Lacteals. Lipids are transported into the lymphatic system via lacteals.

❏❏   **How does soap function?**

Soap has long hydrocarbon tails (i.e., hydrophobic tails) on one side and charged ionic heads on the other side. The hydrocarbon tails are non-polar and therefore dissolve grease. The ionic heads are polar and therefore dissolve in water. Like dissolves/attracts like. Thus, soap has the ability to take up both grease and water.

❏❏   **How does the structural character of a steroid help facilitate its function?**

The lipophilic character of a steroid allows it to pass freely through the cell membrane and into the cell. A steroid then passes directly to the nucleus of the cell and affects the DNA.

ISOMERS

❑❑ **What are isomers ?**

Isomers are compounds that have the same chemical formula but different structures.

❑❑ **List the two major categories of isomers.**

Constitutional (structural) isomers and stereoisomers.

❑❑ **What are constitutional (structural) isomers?**

Constitutional isomers are compounds that have the same atoms connected in a different order.

❑❑ **What are stereoisomers?**

Stereoisomers are compounds that contain atoms in the same order but have different geometry.

❑❑ **What are some types of stereoisomers?**

Enantiomers, diastereomers, and cis-trans diastereomers.

❑❑ **Name the following type of isomers.**

$$CH_3—CH(CH_3)—CH_3 \qquad CH_3—CH_2—CH_2—CH_3$$

These are structural (constitutional) isomers. Count the total carbon and hydrogen molecules and notice that they are equivalent.

❑❑ **What is a chiral carbon?**

A chiral carbon is one that has a plane of symmetry and is not superimposable on its mirror image. This can be most practically identified as a carbon that has four different substituents bound to it.

❑❑   **What type of isomers are the following:**

$$
\begin{array}{ccc}
 & CH_3 & \\
Br\!\!-\!\!\!\!\!- & \!\!\!\!\!-\!\!Cl & \\
H_3C\!\!-\!\!\!\!\!- & \!\!\!\!\!-\!\!H & \\
 & OH &
\end{array}
\qquad
\begin{array}{ccc}
 & CH_3 & \\
Cl\!\!-\!\!\!\!\!- & \!\!\!\!\!-\!\!Br & \\
H\!\!-\!\!\!\!\!- & \!\!\!\!\!-\!\!CH_3 & \\
 & OH &
\end{array}
$$

These are enantiomers, which are a type of stereoisomers. Enantiomers are nonsuperimposable, mirror images. Note the chiral carbon molecules.

❑❑   **What type of isomers are the following:**

$$
\begin{array}{ccc}
 & CH_3 & \\
Br\!\!-\!\!\!\!\!- & \!\!\!\!\!-\!\!Cl & \\
H\!\!-\!\!\!\!\!- & \!\!\!\!\!-\!\!CH_3 & \\
 & OH &
\end{array}
\qquad
\begin{array}{ccc}
 & CH_3 & \\
Cl\!\!-\!\!\!\!\!- & \!\!\!\!\!-\!\!Br & \\
H\!\!-\!\!\!\!\!- & \!\!\!\!\!-\!\!CH_3 & \\
 & OH &
\end{array}
$$

These are diastereomers, which are a type of stereoisomers. Diastereomers are nonsuperimposable, non-mirror images.

❑❑   **What type of isomers are the following:**

$$
\begin{array}{cc}
CH_3\!\!\!\!\!\!\diagdown \qquad \diagup\!\!\!\!\!\!CH_3 \\
C\!\!=\!\!C \\
H\!\!\!\!\!\!\diagup \qquad \diagdown\!\!\!\!\!\!H
\end{array}
\qquad\qquad
\begin{array}{cc}
H\!\!\!\!\!\!\diagdown \qquad \diagup\!\!\!\!\!\!CH_3 \\
C\!\!=\!\!C \\
CH_3\!\!\!\!\!\!\diagup \qquad \diagdown\!\!\!\!\!\!H
\end{array}
$$

The two structures are cis-trans diastereomers, which are a type of stereoisomers.

❏❏ **What type of isomers are the following? Which is more stable?**

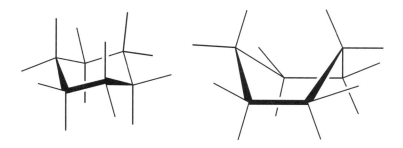

These are conformational isomers. The conformation on the left is the chair form of cyclohexane and on the right is the boat form. The chair form is much more stable than the boat form.

BENZENE

❏❏ **Draw the chemical structure of a benzene molecule.**

❏❏ **What is the term for the configuration of the benzene molecule that gives it unique properties?**

Aromatic.

❏❏ **What does aromatic mean?**

An aromatic compound is a cyclic compound that gains special stability and properties from conjugated pi electrons. The classic aromatic compound is the benzene molecule, but many other conformations can create aromaticity.

❏❏ **Which of the following molecules are aromatic?**

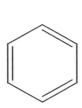 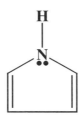 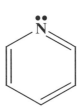

They all are! To determine if a compound is aromatic, apply the "4n +2" rule. Count the number of pi electrons. If they equal a derivative of 4n + 2, then the compound is aromatic. Notice how all three examples have 6 pi electrons and thus fit the rule.

❑❑ **Which of the following molecules are aromatic?**

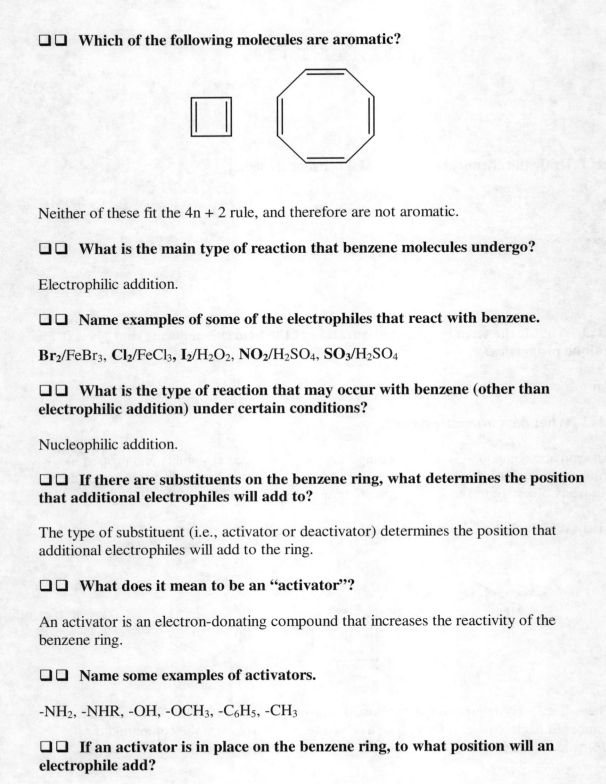

Neither of these fit the 4n + 2 rule, and therefore are not aromatic.

❑❑ **What is the main type of reaction that benzene molecules undergo?**

Electrophilic addition.

❑❑ **Name examples of some of the electrophiles that react with benzene.**

Br_2/$FeBr_3$, Cl_2/$FeCl_3$, I_2/H_2O_2, NO_2/H_2SO_4, SO_3/H_2SO_4

❑❑ **What is the type of reaction that may occur with benzene (other than electrophilic addition) under certain conditions?**

Nucleophilic addition.

❑❑ **If there are substituents on the benzene ring, what determines the position that additional electrophiles will add to?**

The type of substituent (i.e., activator or deactivator) determines the position that additional electrophiles will add to the ring.

❑❑ **What does it mean to be an "activator"?**

An activator is an electron-donating compound that increases the reactivity of the benzene ring.

❑❑ **Name some examples of activators.**

-NH_2, -NHR, -OH, -OCH_3, -C_6H_5, -CH_3

❑❑ **If an activator is in place on the benzene ring, to what position will an electrophile add?**

Activators on the ring cause placement of additional electrophiles to be in either the para or the ortho position. The para position is most favored and electrophiles will add to this position first.

❏❏ **Label the following positions on the benzene molecule:**

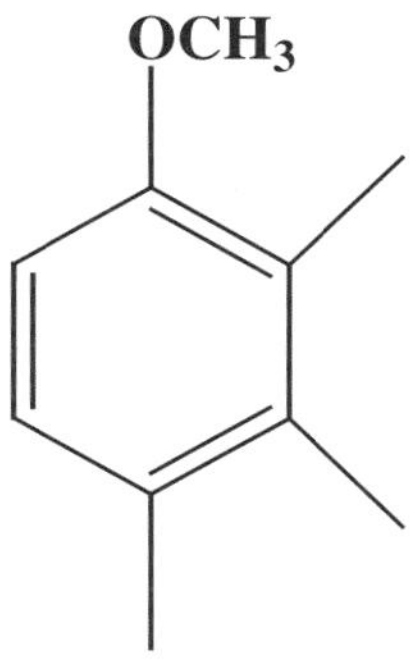

OCH$_3$

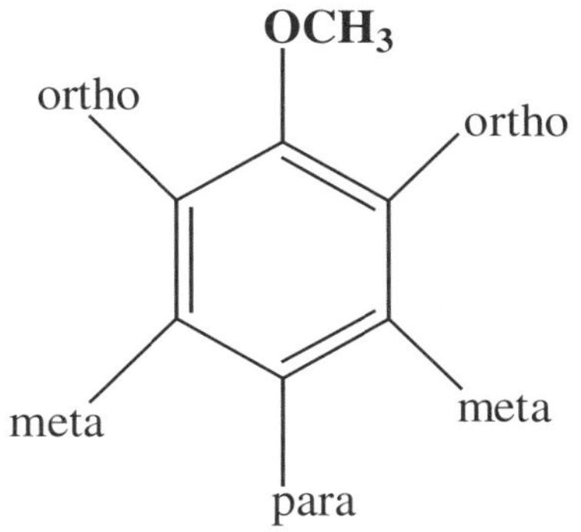

OCH$_3$

ortho   ortho

meta

meta

para

❏❏ **What are the two types of deactivators?**

Deactivators fall into two main categories, namely halogens and non-halogens. This distinction is important, as it determines the placement of an additional electrophile on the benzene ring.

❏❏ **Name some examples of non-halogen deactivators.**

-NO$_2$, -CN, -COOH, -SO$_3$, -CHO

❏❏ **Name the halogen deactivators.**

F, Cl, Br, I

❏❏ **If a deactivator is in place on the ring, to what position will an electrophile add?**

This is a trick question, as you are not given enough information to accurately answer. The determining factor lies in what type of deactivator is on the ring, either a halogen or non-halogen. If a halogen deactivator is in place, an electrophile will add to the para/ortho positions. If a non-halogen deactivator is in place, an electrophile will add to the meta position.

❏❏   **If a halogen deactivator is in place, will an electrophile add to the ortho or the para position first?**

Para first, then ortho.

❏❏   **What is the product of the following reaction?**

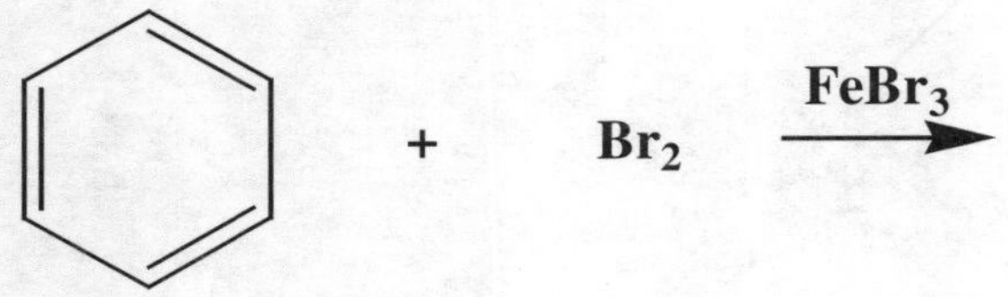

This is an example of electrophilic addition. In this example there are no substituents on the benzene ring, thus the bromide adds to any location on the ring.

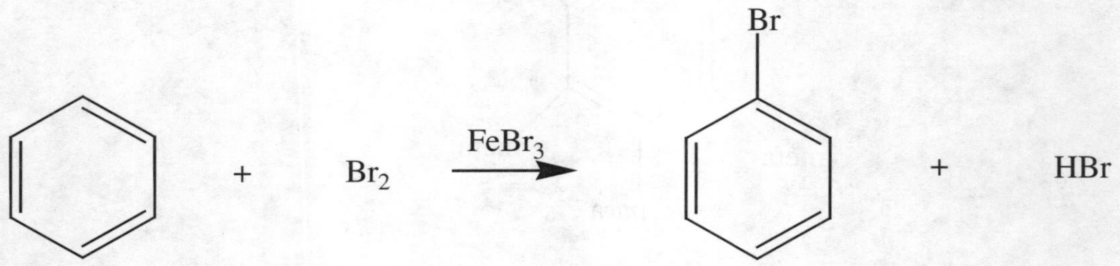

❏❏   **What are the products of the following reaction?**

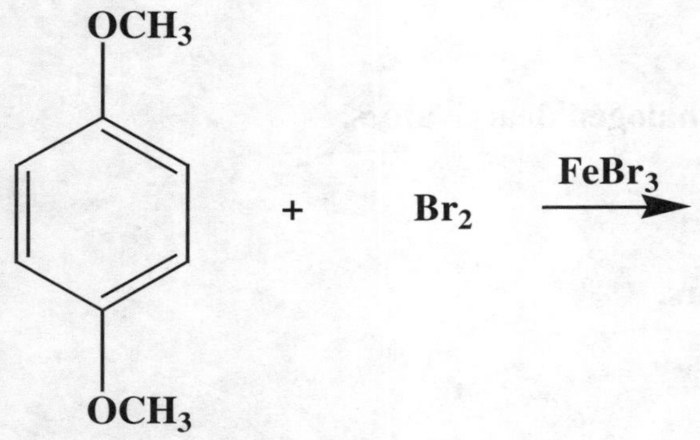

-OCH3 is an activator. Br (the electrophile) will add to the para position if available and then to the ortho position.

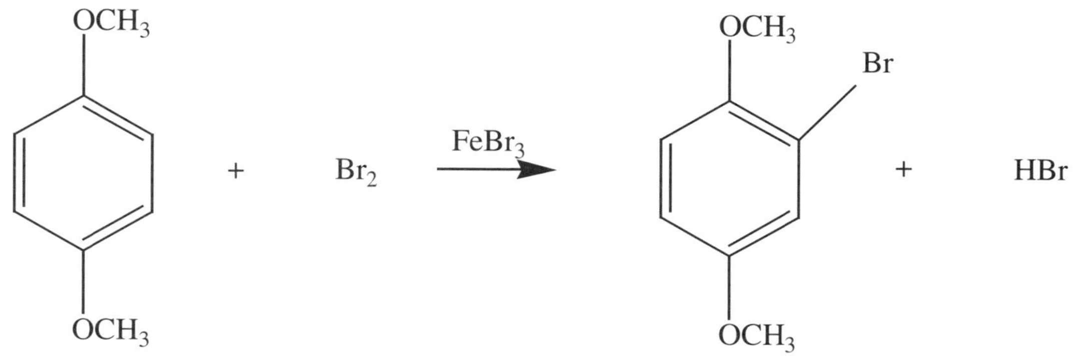

What are the products of the following reaction?

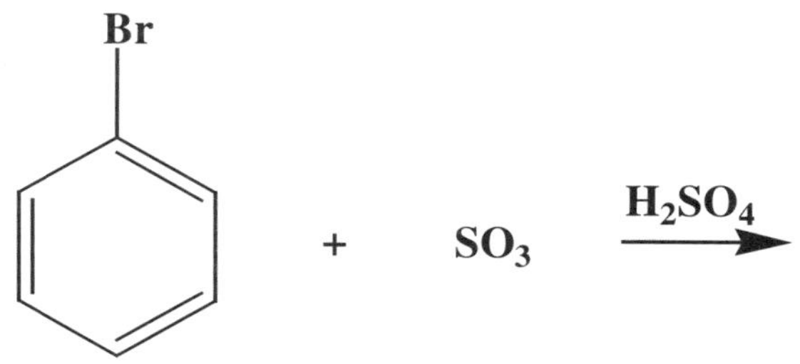

Bromide is a halogen deactivator. Thus, products will end up in the para position first, then the ortho position.

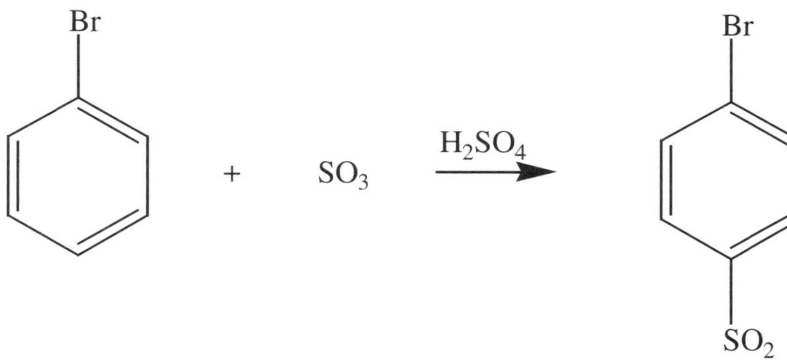

❏❏ **Which reaction will react faster with $Br_2/FeBr_3$?**

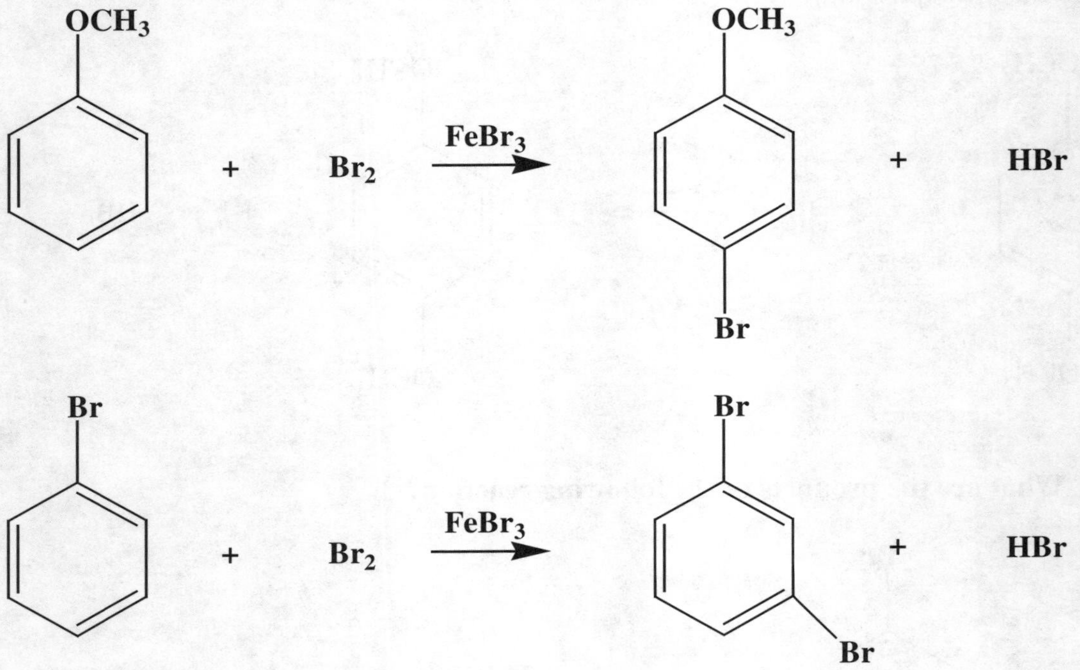

The top reaction will react faster. The substituent in the top reaction is an activator of the benzene ring. Thus, this will be the faster reaction.

❏❏ **What are the products of the following reaction?**

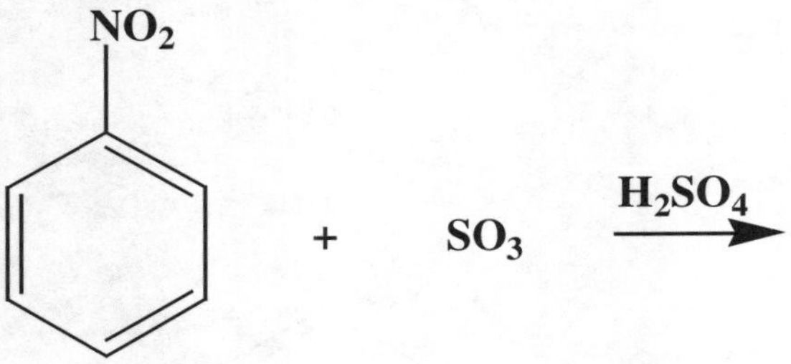

Note that NO_2 is a non-halogen deactivator. Thus, the electrophile (i.e., SO_3) will add to the meta position.

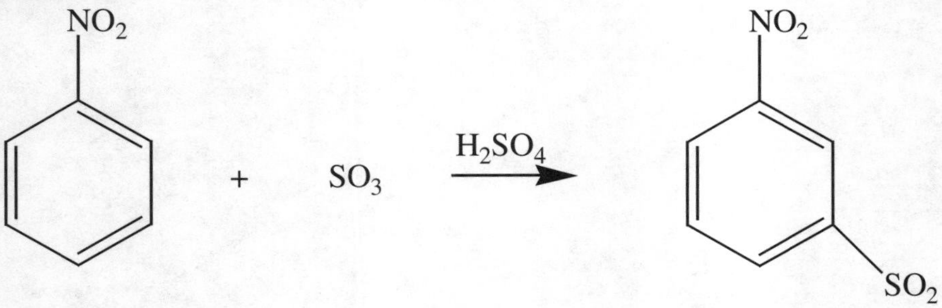

❑❑ **Under what conditions do nucleophilic substitution reactions take place?**

Nucleophilic substitution will occur in the face of an extremely strong base.

❑❑ **What are the products of the following reaction?**

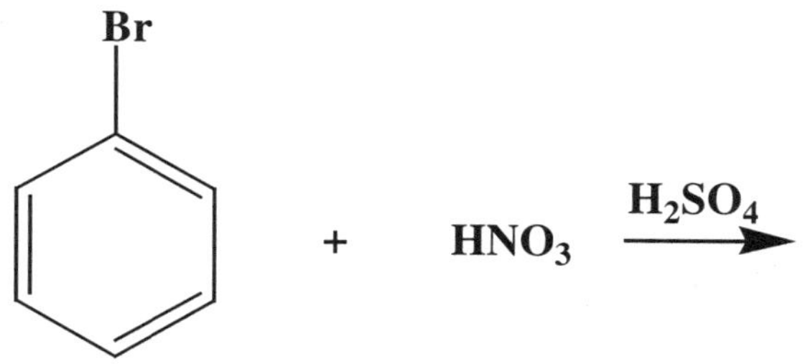

Bromide is a deactivator (halogen) and will result in electrophilic placement to the para and ortho positions. Note that HNO_3 acts as the electrophile and a NO_2 is added to the para position.

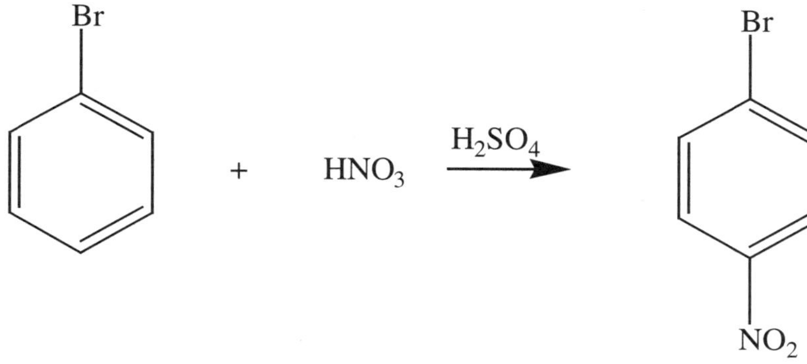

❑❑ **What type of reaction is the following? What are the products?**

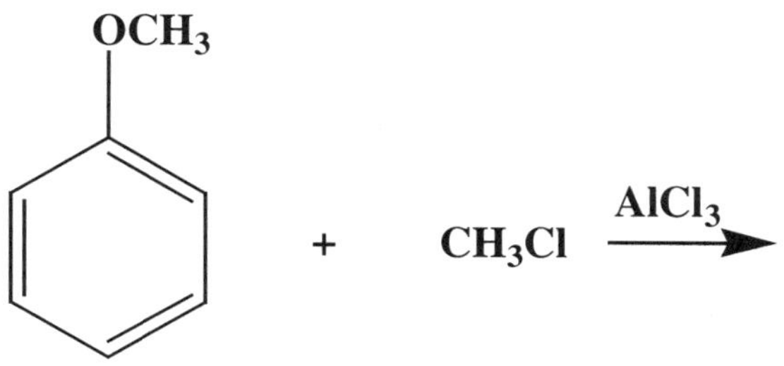

This is a Friedel-Crafts alkylation reaction. The "R" group is added to the benzene ring. In this example, the "R" group is CH_3 and is added to the para position since OCH_3 is an activator.

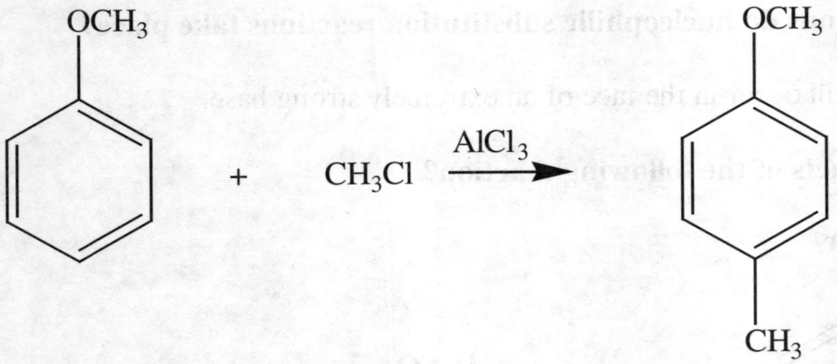

OCH_3 + CH_3Cl $\xrightarrow{\text{AlCl}_3}$ (product: OCH_3 / CH_3)

What is the product of the following reaction?

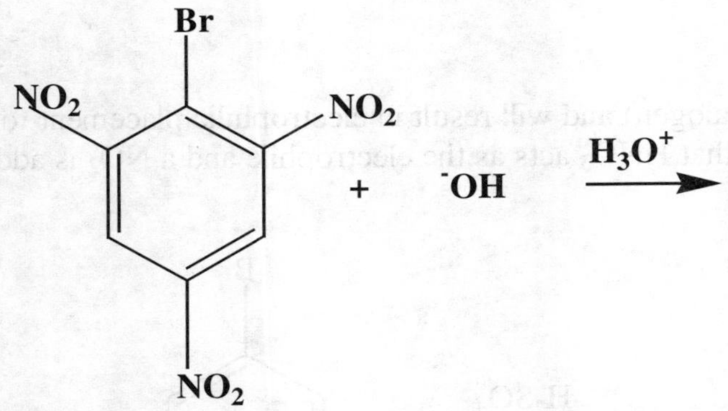

(structure with Br, NO_2 groups) + ^-OH $\xrightarrow{H_3O^+}$

This is an example of a nucleophilic substitution reaction. This reaction occurs in the face of a strong base (-OH). Additionally, note the presence of activating groups in the ortho and para positions.

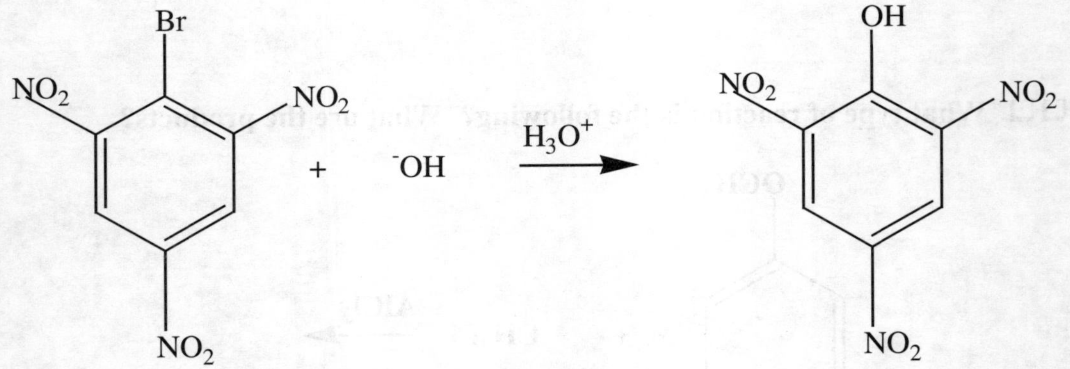

(Br, NO_2 structure) + ^-OH $\xrightarrow{H_3O^+}$ (OH, NO_2 structure)

INFRARED SPECTROSCOPY/NMR

❏❏ **What is the use of infrared spectroscopy (IR) in organic chemistry?**

Certain characteristic absorption patterns are elicited when the functional groups of a molecule absorb infrared radiation. Thus, we can learn which functional groups are present in a molecule by analyzing the infrared spectrum.

❏❏ **What functional group typically has a strong, broad band at a frequency of about 3,300-3,600?**

-OH

❏❏ **What functional group typically has a sharp band at a frequency of about 1,600?**

C=O

❏❏ **What is the use of NMR (nuclear magnetic resonance) spectroscopy?**

NMR spectroscopy can be used to identify the product of a reaction.

❏❏ **How does NMR work?**

^1H and/or ^{13}C are placed in a magnetic field and irradiated. Energy is absorbed and the molecules jump from a lower energy state to a higher energy state. This absorption of energy is displayed as nuclear magnetic resonance (NMR) spectrum.

❏❏ **Is the melting point of a pure substance higher or lower than the melting point of a contaminated specimen?**

A pure substance has a higher melting point than a contaminated substance.

❏❏ **How much will I use organic chemistry in medical school?**

Almost never.

❏❏ **How much will I use organic chemistry as a physician?**

Never.

PHYSICS

GEOMETRY AND MEASUREMENT

❑❑ **What are the circumference and area of a circle compared to its radius r?**

circumference=$2\pi r$, area=πr^2

❑❑ **What are the surface area and volume of a sphere compared to its radius r?**

surface area=$4\pi r^2$, volume=$4\pi r^3/3$

❑❑ **What are the right triangle relations for sine, cosine, and tangent?**

$\sin\theta$ = O/H, $\cos\theta$ = A/H, $\tan\theta$ = O/A

H - hypotenuse
O - opposite side
A - adjacent side

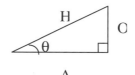

❑❑ **What is the Pythagorean theorem as applied to right triangles?**

$a^2 + b^2 = c^2$

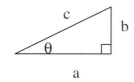

❑❑ **What is another way to express 10^a x 10^b and 10^a / 10^b?**

$10^{(a+b)}$, $10^{(a-b)}$

❑❑ **What are log(ab) and log(a/b)?**

log(a)+log(b), log(a)-log(b)

❑❑ **What is $\log_{10}(10000)$?**

$\log_{10}(10000) = \log_{10}(10^4) = 4$

VECTORS

☐☐ **What is the difference between a scalar and a vector quantity?**

Scalars have magnitude only; vectors have both magnitude and direction.

☐☐ **How does one add vectors?**

The vectors are added "head-to-toe"

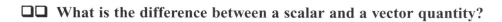

☐☐ **How does one calculate the length of a vector |a| from its horizontal and vertical components a_x and a_y?**

$$a_x^2 + a_y^2 = |a|^2$$

☐☐ **What are the x and y components of a vector a that makes an angle θ with respect to the positive x-axis?**

$$a_x = |a| \cos \theta \ , \ \ a_y = |a| \sin \theta$$

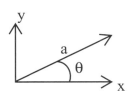

☐☐ **What are the relative lengths of the sides of a 45°-45°-90° triangle?**

$1, 1, \sqrt{2}$

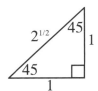

❑❑ **What are the relative lengths of the sides of a 30°-60°-90° triangle?**

$1, \sqrt{3}, 2$

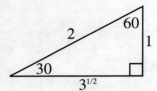

❑❑ **How does one calculate the dot product a•b of two vectors a and b which make an angle θ with each other?**

a•b = |a| |b| cos θ

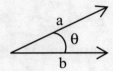

DISPLACEMENT, VELOCITY, AND ACCELERATION

❏❏ **How is the change in a quantity "Δ" defined?**

(Final value) - (initial value)

❏❏ **How does one calculate displacement in the x-direction?**

$\Delta x = x_f - x_i$

❏❏ **How does one calculate average velocity (v_x^{ave}) in the x-direction?**

$v_x^{ave} = \Delta x / \Delta t$

❏❏ **How does one calculate average acceleration (a_x^{ave}) in the x-direction?**

$a_x^{ave} = \Delta v_x / \Delta t$

❏❏ **How is average speed different from average velocity?**

Speed measures distance traveled over time (scalar quantity); velocity measures displacement over time (vector quantity).

❏❏ **If a ball is tossed straight up into the air and allowed to return to its starting point, what is its average velocity in the y-direction (both magnitude and direction)?**

Since the initial and final positions are the same, $\Delta y = y_f - y_i$ and $v_y^{ave} = \Delta y / \Delta t = 0$ (no direction for zero-vector).

❏❏ **If a ball is tossed straight up into the air and allowed to return to its starting point, what is its average acceleration (both magnitude and direction)?**

After the ball is set in motion, the only force that acts on it is gravity, causing it to slow on its ascent, and pick up speed on its downward path. The acceleration is $a_y^{ave} = g = 9.8$ m/s^2 in the downward direction.

❏❏ **How can an object maintain a constant speed and yet still accelerate?**

The object's speed may change directions. An object moving in a circle at a uniform speed is accelerating.

❏❏ **The kinematic equations of motion can only be used under what condition?**

Constant acceleration.

❏❏ **What are the three kinematic equations?**

The kinematic equations describe the relation between position (x), velocity (v) and (constant) acceleration (a) over time (t). They are:

$$\Delta x = v_{ix}t + 1/2\, a_x t^2 \qquad v_{fx} = v_{ix} + a_x t \qquad v_{fx}^2 - v_{ix}^2 = 2a_x \Delta x$$

❏❏ **What is the most common coordinate system applied to problems?**

Positive x pointing to "right", positive y pointing "up."

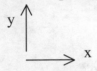

❏❏ **Using the most common coordinate system, what would a negative v_y imply? A negative v_x?**

Downward motion; motion to the "left".

❏❏ **If the coordinate system was changed so that the positive y-axis pointed down, what direction would a positive v_y imply?**

Down.

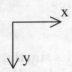

❏❏ **Why is the origin (intersection of x- and y-axes) of the coordinate system important?**

It defines the point where x=0 and y=0. All other values of x and y are measured from it.

❏❏ **Is there a correct spot to place the coordinate system when solving problems?**

No. One may place the coordinate system anywhere - choose a spot that will simplify calculations.

❏❏ **If v_x and a_x have opposite signs, what is happening?**

The object is decelerating (slowing down).

❏❏ **If an object is thrown horizontally off a cliff with velocity v_o, what is its velocity and acceleration in the x-direction just before it hits the ground (neglecting air friction)?**

After the ball is thrown, no force acts on it in the horizontal direction. Hence its horizontal acceleration is zero. Since $a_x = 0$, $v_{fx} = v_o + 0(t) = v_o$

❏❏ **If an object is thrown straight up, how does the v_y change on the upward path, the top of the flight, and the downward path (assuming the most common coordinate system)?**

v_y is positive on the way up, zero at the top, and negative on the way down.

❏❏ **If an object is thrown straight up, how does the a_y change on the upward path, the top of the flight, and the downward path (assuming most common coordinate system)?**

a_y is always $-g$ (g = gravitational constant = 9.8 m/s^2).

❏❏ **What is the only difference in velocity and acceleration between a ball thrown straight up, and a ball thrown to the same height from one person to another (projectile)?**

The latter has a constant velocity in the x-direction. The v_y and a_y are the same in both examples.

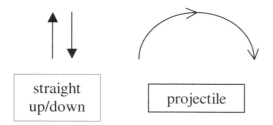

| straight up/down | projectile |

❏❏ **In centripetal acceleration, what is the shape of the motion and the relation of v to this motion?**

The motion is circular, and v is the velocity tangent to the circle (the velocity vector would touch the circle at only one point).

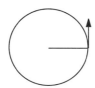

❑❑   **What is the formula for and the unit of centripetal acceleration a_c?**

$a_c = v^2/r$; m/s^2 where v = velocity (m/s) and r = radius of the circular path (m).

FORCE AND WORK

❏❏ **What is Newton's first law of motion?**

A body will move at a constant velocity unless a net force acts.

❏❏ **Is a satellite orbiting the earth with a constant speed experiencing a net force?**

Yes, because the velocity is not constant; its direction is changing.

❏❏ **Is an object dropping at its terminal velocity (constant speed) experiencing a net force? If so, what force(s)?**

No - forces from gravity and air resistance are equal and opposite. The net force is zero and the velocity is constant.

❏❏ **What is Newton's second law of motion and the formula associated with it?**

The acceleration of an object is proportional to the net force acting on it. (F = ma where F = force, m = mass, a = acceleration).

❏❏ **What is the metric unit of force?**

Newton (N) = kg m/s^2

❏❏ **What kind of force is experienced by an orbiting satellite and what is the formula associated with it?**

Centripetal force (F_c). $F_c = ma_c = mv^2/r$ (m= mass [kg], a_c= centripetal acceleration, v = velocity [m/s], and r = radius of the circular path [m]).

❏❏ **What is the formula for the force we associate with weight?**

W = mg (g = gravitational constant [9.8 m/s^2]).

❏❏ **What is Newton's third law of motion?**

Each action elicits an equal and opposite reaction.

❏❏ **What is a normal force?**

A force that acts perpendicular to a contact surface.

❑❑ **For a stationary block on a frictionless inclined plane, what forces act on the block, and in which direction do they act?**

Gravity acts straight down; a normal force is exerted by the inclined plane perpendicular to the surface.

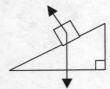

❑❑ **How does the frictional force change if the same object is placed on a side with more surface area?**

It doesn't change - provided the frictional force really is proportional to the normal force, and no "sticky" substance has been applied.

❑❑ **What is the most common coordinate system used for inclined plane problems?**

X-axis pointed along slope, parallel to plane; y-axis perpendicular to slope, parallel to normal force.

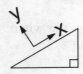

❑❑ **Without friction, what is the direction of the net force exerted on a block on an inclined plane?**

Down the slope.

❑❑ **In what direction does friction act?**

It acts in the opposite direction of motion.

❑❑ **What is the formula for calculating the force of friction (F_f)?**

$F_f = \mu N$ where N is the normal force and μ is the coefficient of friction.

❑❑ **What is the difference between static and kinetic friction?**

Static friction occurs between stationary objects and uses the coefficient of static friction μ_s; kinetic friction occurs between objects in motion and uses the coefficient of kinetic friction μ_k.

❏❏ **Which is typically larger, μ_s or μ_k?**

μ_s

❏❏ **If an inclined plane makes an angle θ with respect to the horizontal, what are the components of weight and the normal force, using an inclined plane coordinate system?**

$W_x = mg\sin\theta$, $N_x = 0$, $W_y = mg\cos\theta = -N_y$

❏❏ **When a block slides down an inclined plane, what forces do work, and what kind of work do they do?**

Friction - does negative work, because the force opposes the direction of displacement.
Normal - does no work, because it is perpendicular to the displacement.
Gravity - the component parallel to the plane does positive work. The component
           perpendicular to the plane does none.

❏❏ **As a block slides down a frictionless inclined plane, how does the final kinetic energy of the block at the bottom of the plane compare with the initial potential energy? How does friction change this?**

For a frictionless plane, the final kinetic energy would equal the initial potential energy, because only conservative forces acted. If friction is present, the final kinetic energy would be less than the initial potential energy. The energy losses are converted to thermal energy.

❏❏ **What is the formula for Hooke's law (force exerted by a spring)? What are the units for each term?**

$F = -kx$ where F is the force (in N), x is the displacement from equilibrium position (in m), and k is the spring constant (N/m).

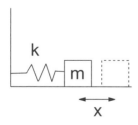

❏❏ **What does the negative sign in Hooke's law indicate?**

The force acts in the opposite direction of the displacement (if a spring is compressed to the left, it will push to the right, and vice versa).

❑❑ **What is the formula for work done by a constant force?**

Work = F•d = |F| |d| cos θ where θ is the angle between the force F and the displacement d. Work is done only when the applied force is in the direction of the displacement. In this case, only the force component (F cos θ) is applied in the direction of the displacement d.

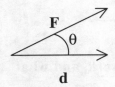

❑❑ **What is the metric unit of work?**

joule (j) = kg m^2 / s^2

❑❑ **How does one calculate the work done by a non-constant force?**

It is the area under a F_x vs. x curve.

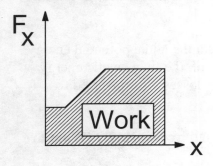

❑❑ **What is the work done on a spring when it is compressed or stretched a distance x?**

Work = 1/2 kx^2

❑❑ **What work is done by a pillar supporting a roof?**

None - the pillar exerts a force, but does not displace the roof.

❑❑ **When can work be negative?**

When the force is exerted in a direction opposing the object's motion; kinetic friction always involves negative work.

❑❑ **What is the formula for calculating average power (P$_{ave}$), and the metric unit for power?**

P$_{ave}$ = W/Δt ; watt (w) = joules (j)/second (s) where W is the work done over time t.

❑❑ **Estimate how many Calories (kcal) a 60-watt light bulb consumes in an hour (1 cal = 4.18 j) ?**

Total energy used = Power * Δt = 60 joules/s (1 hr) (3600s/hr) ~ 250000 j
    250000 j (1 cal/4.2 j) ~ 60000 cal = 60 kcal

ENERGY AND MOMENTUM CONSERVATION

❑❑ **What is the formula for kinetic energy (K)?**

$K = 1/2\ mv^2$ where m = mass (kg) and v = velocity (m/s).

❑❑ **If g is constant, how does one calculate gravitational potential energy (U_{grav})?**

U_{grav} = mgh where m = mass (kg), g = gravitational constant ($9.8\ m/s^2$), h = height.

❑❑ **If g is not constant, how does one calculate gravitational potential energy?**

U_{grav} = -G mM_e/r (M_e is the mass of the earth, r is the distance from the object to the center of the earth, G = univeral gravitational constant [$7 \times 10^{-11}\ n\cdot m^2/kg^2$])).

❑❑ **Another way to express g is $g=GM/r^2$. Assuming $g_{earth} = 10\ m/s^2$, what would g be for a planet with twice the mass of earth and half the radius?**

$g'/g = (M'/M)(r/r')^2 = (2)(2)^2 = 8$. $g' = 8g = 80\ m/s^2$.

❑❑ **What is the elastic potential energy (U_{elas}) of a compressed or stretched spring?**

$U_{elas} = 1/2\ kx^2$ (k = spring constant [N/m], x = displacement).

❑❑ **What is the difference between mechanical energy and internal energy?**

Mechanical energy is the sum of kinetic and potential energy and depends on motion and position; internal energy represents "hidden" forms of energy like thermal energy and chemical bonds.

❑❑ **How does one define a system?**

A group of objects is selected and an imaginary boundary is drawn separating the system (inside) from the environment (outside).

❑❑ **When is energy conserved in a system?**

When no net work is done on the system by the environment.

❏❏ **What is the formula for linear momentum (p)? What are the units?**

p = mv where m = mass (kg) and v = velocity (m/s).

❏❏ **When is momentum conserved in a system?**

When no net force is exerted on the system by the environment.

❏❏ **In an inelastic collision, which quantity is conserved?**

Momentum, but not kinetic energy.

❏❏ **Two identical pucks traveling in opposite directions on a frictionless surface collide and stick together. If one puck initially has twice the velocity v of the other, what is the final velocity of the two pucks?**

This is an inelastic collision. Therefore, momentum is conserved and $p_i = p_f$ (p_i = initial momentum and p_f = final momentum). The initial momentum is p_i= mv + m(-2v) and the final momentum is p_f= $2mv_f$. Equating the two yields -mv=$2mv_f$, so v_f = -v/2. (The velocity is half that of the slower puck, and in the opposite direction.)

❏❏ **How does one calculate the center of mass for three objects with masses m_1,m_2,m_3 and x-coordinates x_1,x_2,x_3?**

$x_{cm} = (m_1*x_1 + m_2*x_2 + m_3*x_3) / (m_1 + m_2 + m_3) = (\Sigma\ m_i*x_i) / (\Sigma\ m_i)$

❏❏ **How does the center of mass relate to the force of gravity?**

Gravity can be thought to act on a body's center of mass (the force vector originates there).

❏❏ **Why is one allowed to pick any reference point measuring the height h in U_{grav}?**

Because changes in potential energy ΔU_{grav} are most important, and ΔU_{grav} = mgΔh does not depend on the reference point for h (provided g remains constant).

❏❏ **If energy is being conserved in a system and the kinetic energy increases, what happens to the potential energy?**

The potential energy decreases by the same amount.

❏❏ **What is the difference between a conservative and a non-conservative force?**

Conservative forces do not change the mechanical energy (K+U) of a system, while a non-conservative force (friction) decreases the mechanical energy.

ROTATIONAL MOTION AND GRAVITATION

❑❑ **How does one calculate the length of an arc?**

$s = r \, \Delta\theta$ where s is the arc length, r is the radius and $\Delta\theta$ is the angle in radians.

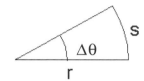

❑❑ **How does one calculate torque?**

$T = r \times F = |r| \, |F| \sin\theta$ where r is the distance from pivot point to applied force F, and θ is the angle between force and lever arm.

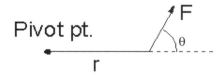

❑❑ **What are the units of torque?**

Newton-meter (Nm) = $kg \, m^2/s^2$ (same as joule)

❑❑ **How does one calculate average angular velocity (ω_{ave}) and what are its units?**

$\omega_{ave} = \Delta\theta / \Delta t$; rads/s

❑❑ **How does one calculate average angular acceleration (α_{ave}) and what are its units?**

$\alpha_{ave} = \Delta\omega / \Delta t$; rads/s^2

❑❑ **How does one convert angular velocity (ω) and acceleration (α) to linear (tangential) velocity and acceleration?**

Multiply by radius r of the circular motion: $v = \omega r$, $a = \alpha r$

❑❑ **How does one assign the direction of a rotational vector like ω, α, or torque?**

Right hand rule. Curl fingers in direction of motion (either clockwise or counterclockwise); thumb will point in direction of vector.

❑❑ **Instead of mass, what quantity is used to indicate inertia in rotational motion?**

Rotational inertia: $I = mr^2$; the r^2 term indicates that bodies are harder to rotate (have more inertia) when they are farther from the axis of rotation.

❑❑ **What is the rotational version of Newton's second law?**

$T = I\alpha$ (compare to $F = ma$). The angular acceleration (α) is proportional to the net torque (T).

❑❑ **What are the rotational kinematic equations, and under what condition do they apply?**

$\Delta\theta = \omega_i t + 1/2 \; \alpha t^2$ $\omega_f = \omega_i + \alpha t$ $\omega_f^2 - \omega_i^2 = 2\alpha\Delta\theta$; constant angular acceleration α

❑❑ **How does one calculate rotational kinetic energy?**

$K_{rot} = 1/2 \; I\omega^2$ (I = rotational inertia and ω = angular velocity).

❑❑ **If a sphere of mass M is rolling at a velocity v and has rotational inertia 2/5 Mr^2, what is its total kinetic energy?**

$K_{tot} = K_{lin} + K_{rot} = 1/2 \; Mv^2 + 1/2 \; (2/5 \; Mr^2) \; (v/r)^2 = 1/2 \; Mv^2 + 1/5 \; Mv^2 = 7/10 \; Mv^2$

❑❑ **What is the formula for angular momentum (L)?**

$L = I\omega$ (compare to $p = mv$).

❑❑ **When does a system conserve angular momentum?**

When no net torque acts on the system; $T_{clockwise} = T_{counterclockwise}$

❑❑ **What are the two conditions for a system to be in equilibrium?**

Translational equilibrium - no net force acts; rotational equilibrium - no net torque acts.

❏❏ **When torques are calculated, where should the pivot point be placed?**

Any place. Put it in a spot that simplifies calculations - if it coincides with the location of an applied force, the torque of that force will be zero.

❏❏ **What is the formula for Newton's law of gravitation?**

$F = G\, m_1 m_2 / r^2$ where m_1 and m_2 are the masses (in kg), r is the distance (in m) between the objects' centers of mass, and G is the universal gravitational constant.

❏❏ **Looking at Newton's law of gravitation, what are the units of G?**

Nm^2/kg^2

FLUIDS

❑❑ **What is the definition of pressure and its units?**

Pressure = Force/Area or P = F/A; Pascal (Pa) = n/m^2.

❑❑ **What is the definition of density and its metric units?**

ρ = m/V = mass/volume; g/cm^3 or g/ml.

❑❑ **What is the density of water at 25° C?**

ρ_{water} = 1 g/ml = 1 g/cm^3.

❑❑ **What is specific gravity?**

The ratio of a liquid's density compared to the density of water. Specific gravity = ρ/ρ_{water}

❑❑ **If a piece of Styrofoam has 1/3 the density of water, what fraction of it is hidden below the surface?**

1/3. Why is this true? (Note - it's easier to calculate the fraction submerged rather than the fraction that floats.) If one takes the total volume as V and the submerged volume as V_1 , then the buoyant force provided by the displaced water is $F_{buoyant} = m_{sty}g = (\rho_{sty}V)g = m_{water}g=(\rho_{water}V_1)g$.   This works out to $V_1/V = \rho_{sty}/\rho_{water} = 1/3$.

❑❑ **What is hydrostatic pressure caused by and how does one calculate it?**

It is the pressure exerted by a fluid at rest. P_{hydro} = ρgh where h is the height of the column of fluid.

❑❑ **What is Bernoulli's equation? How does it relate to the pressure (p) of a moving fluid?**

$p_1 + 1/2\rho v_1^2 + \rho gh_1 = p_2 + 1/2\rho v_2^2 + \rho gh_2$ (The pressure of a fluid depends on its velocity and position; generally, the faster a fluid flows, the less pressure it exerts on objects around it.)

❑❑ How does Bernoulli's equation account for the lift generated by an airplane wing?

Air flows more rapidly over the top of the wing (v_1) than the bottom (v_2). In accordance with Bernoulli's equation, since $v_1 > v_2$, it follows that $p_1 < p_2$. This difference in pressure causes lift.

❑❑ What is Pascal's principle?

If a fluid is enclosed, a change in pressure is transmitted to all parts of the fluid. As an equation, this would read $F_1/A_1 = F_2/A_2$

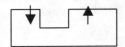

❑❑ How does one calculate the flow rate R of fluid through a channel with given cross-sectional area A?

$R = Av$ (in liters/s or cm^3/s) where v is the velocity of the fluid.

❑❑ If the flow rate through all parts of a channel is constant, how does the speed of the fluid change when it encounters a cross-sectional area reduced by a factor of 4?

Since R is constant, the velocity v increases by a factor of 4.

❑❑ What is the buoyant force and how is it calculated?

When an object displaces a fluid (like water), it experiences an upward force equal to the weight of the fluid displaced. $F_{buoy} = V_{disp} \rho g$ ($V_{disp} \rho$ is the mass of the displaced fluid).

PERIODIC MOTION AND WAVES

❑❑ **What is periodic motion? How is simple harmonic motion (SHM) different?**

Periodic motion is any motion that repeats itself. SHM can be plotted over time as a sine or cosine curve.

❑❑ **What type of force is responsible for simple harmonic motion? Give two examples.**

A force which is proportional to displacement. A spring system and a small-angle simple pendulum.

❑❑ **What constitutes a single "period"?**

The time required for one complete oscillation.

❑❑ **How is frequency related to period, and what is the unit of frequency?**

$f = 1/T$; Hertz (Hz or hz) $= 1/s$. A Hertz is one cycle per second.

❑❑ **How does one represent simple harmonic motion along the x-axis with a sine wave?**

$x(t) = x_o \sin(\omega t + \phi)$

❑❑ **In the expression for simple harmonic motion, what do x_o, ω and ϕ represent?**

x_o is the maximum displacement (also known as the amplitude), ω is the angular frequency and is related to the period T by $\omega = 2\pi/T$ (rads/s) and ϕ is a phase that can be used to adjust the starting point at $t = 0$.

❑❑ **What is the sinusoidal description of a traveling wave?**

$y(x,t) = x_o \sin(\omega t + kx)$

❑❑ **What quantities are represented by x_o, ω, k?**

x_o ,is the amplitude, $\omega = 2\pi/T$ is the angular frequency, $k = 2\pi/\lambda$ is the wavenumber (and λ is the wavelength).

❑❑ **What do mechanical waves (like sound) require which light does not?**

A material medium in which to travel.

❑❑ **What is the difference between a transverse wave (like light) and a longitudinal wave (like sound)?**

In transverse waves, the displacement is perpendicular to the direction of the wave, while in longitudinal waves, the displacement is back and forth along the same direction as the wave.

❑❑ **How does one calculate the velocity of a wave?**

$v = \lambda / T = f\lambda$ where f = frequency and λ = wavelength.

❑❑ **What is destructive interference? constructive interference?**

The amplitudes of two waves add together to form a smaller (destructive) or a larger (constructive) amplitude.

❑❑ **What is the wavelength of the fundamental frequency for a string of length L clamped at both ends?**

$\lambda = 2L$

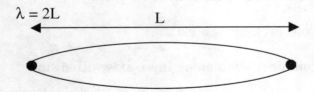

❑❑ **How does the second harmonic for a clamped string compare in wavelength and frequency to the fundamental harmonic?**

$f' = 2f.$ $\lambda = L$

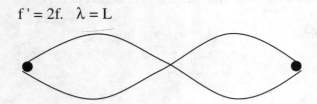

❑❑ **What is the difference between a node and an antinode?**

An antinode is a place of maximum displacement in a standing wave, while a node is a place of minimum displacement.

❑❑ **What is the fundamental wavelength for an open pipe of length L? Where are the nodes and antinodes?**

$\lambda = 4L$

L

antinode : node

❑❑ **What is the formula for intensity?**

I = Power / Area (watts/m^2)

❑❑ **How does one calculate sound intensity in decibels?**

$I(db) = 10 \log(I/I_o)$ where $I_o = 10^{-14}$ w/cm^2

❑❑ **If two nearby sound frequencies are present, what does the listener hear?**

Beats; # beats = $f_2 - f_1$

❑❑ **How does the power of a wave depend on its amplitude?**

The power is proportional to the square of the amplitude.

❑❑ **What happens to the frequency and wavelength of a sound if the source and observer are moving apart from each other?**

The frequency decreases while the wavelength increases.

❑❑ **How does one calculate the Doppler shift of a frequency for a moving source or moving observer?**

$f = f_o (v_{sound} +/- v_{obs}) / (v_{sound} +/- v_{source})$ where f_o is the original frequency and f is the shifted frequency. To determine the appropriate signs, remember that if the source moves toward the observer, or vice versa, the frequency should increase. Therefore, if the source moves toward the observer, the sign for v_{source} is (-). If the observer moves toward the source, the sign for v_{obs} is (+).

208

THERMODYNAMICS AND TEMPERATURE

❑❑ **How does one convert from Celsius (T_c) to Kelvin (T_k)?**

$T_k = T_c + 273$ (In the Kelvin scale, temperature can never be negative.)

❑❑ **How much energy is in one calorie?**

4.187 joules; enough to raise the temperature of 1 g of water $1^\circ C$ at room temperature.

❑❑ **How much energy is in one Calorie of food?**

1 Calorie = 1000 calories = 4187 j.

❑❑ **What is the formula for the specific heat of a material?**

$Q = cm(T_f - T_i)$ where c is the specific heat (in $j/g\,^\circ C$ or $cal/g\,^\circ C$) and Q is the energy required to change the temperature of mass m (in g) from T_i to T_f.

❑❑ **What happens to the temperature of a substance while it changes phase?**

The temperature remains constant.

❑❑ **What is the formula for the heat of transformation?**

$Q = L\,m$ where L is the heat of transformation (in j/g or cal/g) and Q is the amount of energy required to change mass m (in g) from one phase to another (like liquid to gas).

❑❑ **What is implied by a negative heat of transformation? Give an example.**

Energy is released during the transformation, rather than absorbed. The condensation of water vapor to liquid, and the freezing of water to ice are two examples.

❑❑ **What are the three heat transfer mechanisms?**

Conduction - occurs when two objects are in contact with each other. Convection - heated fluid carries both matter and energy away. Radiation - electromagnetic waves carry energy from one object to another (sun to earth).

❑❑ **If two panes of glass in a house window are separated by a thin evacuated region, what is the only heating mechanism that can still warm the house from the outside?**

Radiative heating. Electromagnetic waves (like light) do not require a medium (like air) in order to travel, and can be absorbed by objects in the house.

❑❑ **What is the formula for the first law of thermodynamics?**

$\Delta E = Q - W$ (where E is the total energy of the system, Q is a heat transfer from the environment to the system, and W is work done by the system on the environment).

❑❑ **For gases at constant pressure, what is the work done during expansion or contraction?**

$W = P\Delta V$ (where ΔV is the change in volume).

❑❑ **What is the second law of thermodynamics?**

The total entropy (disorder) cannot decrease for a natural process.

❑❑ **When one measures the efficiency of a process, how does one calculate it?**

efficiency = $work_{out}$ / $work_{in}$ or efficiency = $power_{out}$ / $power_{in}$

❑❑ **What is the efficiency of a 2-horsepower engine that lifts 20 kg at 2 m/s (1hp = 746 w, and assume $g=10m/s^2$)?**

For constant velocity, P_{out} = Fv = mgv = $(20kg)(10 m/s^2)(2 m/s)$ = 400 w.
P_{in} = 2 hp(746 w/hp) ~ 1500 w. Efficiency = P_{out}/P_{in} = 400/1500 ~27%.

❑❑ **What is the ideal gas law formula?**

$PV = nRT$

❑❑ **How is temperature related to energy?**

The temperature (in K) of an object is proportional to the average kinetic energy of its particles. For example, K_{ave} = 3/2 kT for a monatomic gas, where k is the Boltzmann constant (in j/K).

❑❑ **How do the speeds of a water molecule (H_2O) and a carbon dioxide molecule (CO_2) compare at the same temperature?**

On average the kinetic energy is the same. Since CO_2 has the larger mass (44 u compared to 18 u for water), it will have the smaller speed.

ELECTRIC FIELD AND ELECTRIC POTENTIAL

❑❑ **What is Coulomb's law for the electrostatic force between two charges q_1 and q_2?**

$F = kq_1q_2/r^2$ where r is the distance between the charges and k is a constant (different from the Boltzmann constant).

❑❑ **What are the units of k in Coulomb's law?**

Nm^2/c^2 where c = coulombs

❑❑ **How is the electric field E defined?**

It is the (vector) force experienced by a positive test charge. $E = F/q_o$ (unit = N/c)

❑❑ **Where do electric field lines originate and end?**

Electric field lines originate on positive charges and end on negative charges.

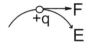

❑❑ **If a field line is curved, how is one to interpret the direction of the force experienced by the test charge?**

The force should act tangent to (intersect at one point) the field line.

❑❑ **How is the intensity of an electric field represented in a drawing?**

The higher the density of field lines, the more intense the electric field.

❏❏ **How does one calculate the force (F) experienced by a charge (q) in an electric field (E)?**

$F = qE$

❏❏ **What is the electric field between two parallel plates 2 cm apart with a potential difference of 10 volts?**

Between parallel plates the field is assumed to be uniform with $E = V/d = 10\ V/0.02\ m = 500\ V/m$ or $500\ N/c$.

❏❏ **What is the unit of charge?**

coulomb $= 6.24 \times 10^{18}\ e^-$

❏❏ **How is the electric potential defined?**

$V = U/q_o$ in volts (V) = joule/coulomb (j/c) where U is the electric potential energy.

❏❏ **What has happened to a charge if its electric potential increases ($\Delta V > 0$)?**

Its electric potential energy has increased.

❏❏ **How does one calculate the potential due to a point charge q?**

$V_{pt\ chg} = kq / r$

❏❏ **As one goes to larger and larger distances from a point charge, what happens to the electric potential $V_{pt\ chg}$ due to that charge?**

It goes to zero.

❏❏ **How is the electric potential of a point charge $V_{pt\ chg}$ related to the work done on other charges?**

The potential is the amount of work (per unit charge) required to bring another charge from infinity to a distance r from the point charge.

❏❏ **What is an electron-volt?**

The amount of energy acquired by an electron as it is accelerated across a potential difference of 1V. 1 eV= (1 e⁻)*(1 V) = (1.6x10⁻¹⁹ C)*(1 j/C) = 1.6x10⁻¹⁹ j. It serves as a convenient small unit of energy.

❏❏ **What would be the electric potential energy of a proton sitting at a potential of +5 V?**

$U = qV = (+1e^-)(5V) = 5\ eV$

❑❑ **If an electron at rest started from an electrode at -5V and traveled to an electrode at +5V, what would be the changes in its kinetic and potential energies?**

$\Delta U = q\Delta V = (-1e^-)(+5V - (-5V)) = -10$ eV; the potential energy decreased by 10 eV
$\Delta E = \Delta U + \Delta K = 0$, so $\Delta K = -\Delta U = 10$ eV; the kinetic energy increased by 10 eV

❑❑ **What is the electric potential of "ground"?**

0 V

❑❑ **How would one calculate the electric field or electric potential of three charges q1,q2,q3?**

The total electric field would be the vector sum of the individual electric fields E_1, E_2, E_3. The total electric potential would be the scalar sum of the individual electric potentials V_1, V_2, V_3.

ELECTRIC CIRCUITS

❑❑ **What is the definition of capacitance and its unit?**

$C = Q/V$; farad (F) = coulomb/volt (c/V).

❑❑ **What is the formula for the energy stored in a capacitor?**

$U = 1/2 \, CV^2$

❑❑ **If $1/c = 1/a + 1/b$, what is a simple way to calculate c?**

$c = a*b/(a+b)$

❑❑ **If a set of capacitors is hooked up in series, what is the total capacitance (C_{tot})?**

$1/C_{tot} = 1/C_1 + 1/C_2 + \dots$

❑❑ **If a set of capacitors is hooked up in parallel, what is the total capacitance?**

$C_{tot} = C_1 + C_2 + \dots$

❑❑ **The capacitance of a parallel plate capacitor can be changed by inserting a material between the plates with a different dielectric constant κ. What is the formula for this change?**

$C' = \kappa C$ (the dielectric constant for vacuum is 1, for air ~1) where C and C' are the old and new capacitances, respectively.

❑❑ **What is a primary function for capacitors?**

The storage of charge. In a camera flash, the charge is rapidly released during the flash. In electronic circuits, capacitors can act as a buffer, temporarily absorbing excess charge.

❑❑ **What is a resistor?**

Any object that resists the flow of current in a circuit.

❑❑ **What is the definition of current and its unit?**

$I = q/t$;   Ampere (A) = 1 coulomb/second (c/s)   The amount of charge that passes a given point in a circuit over time.

❏❏ **What is Ohm's law for resistors?**

R = V / I where R = resistance (ohms, Ω), V = voltage (volts), and I = current (amperes).

❏❏ **Why does one refer to a "potential drop" across a resistor?**

The charge passing through a resistor experiences a decrease in electric potential $\Delta V = IR$.

❏❏ **How is the resistance of a wire related to its resistivity ρ?**

$R = \rho L / A$ where ρ is the resistivity of the material, L is the length, and A is the cross-sectional area.

❏❏ **How would the resistivities of conductors compare to that of insulators?**

The resistivity of conductors is low, while the resistivity of insulators is high.

❏❏ **How much power does a resistor consume?**

$P = VI = I^2R = V^2R$

❏❏ **What is the emf of a battery?**

emf (electromotive force) is the potential difference (ΔV) supplied by a battery in an open circuit.

❏❏ **What is the internal resistance of a battery r_{int} and how does it relate to the battery's emf?**

r_{int} is the battery's effective resistance to the flow of charge; since this resistance is in series with any circuit connected to the battery, it is responsible for a small loss of potential ΔV_{int}. The voltage delivered to the circuit is less than the emf. $\varepsilon = \Delta V_{int} + \Delta V_{circuit}$

❏❏ **If resistors are arranged in series, what is the total resistance (R_{tot})?**

$R_{tot} = R_1 + R_2 + \ldots$

❏❏ **If resistors are arranged in parallel, what is the total resistance?**

$1/R_{tot} = 1/R_1 + 1/R_2 + \ldots$

❏❏ **If batteries are arranged in series, what is the total emf?**

$\varepsilon_{tot} = \varepsilon_1 + \varepsilon_2 + \ldots$

❑❑ **What is the junction rule for DC (direct current) circuits?**

The sum of currents entering a junction must equal the sum of currents leaving a junction; $i_{in} = i_{out}$

❑❑ **What is the loop rule for DC circuits?**

The sum of potential drops about a loop must equal zero.

❑❑ **How is "conventional current" defined?**

As a flow of positive charge (even though the physical entities that move are generally electrons).

❑❑ **If a single battery is used in a circuit, from which terminal does conventional current originate?**

Since conventional current is a flow of positive charge, the "large" line representing the positive terminal of the battery is the origin of the current.

positive | | -
⊥

❑❑ **What generally happens to the resistance of an object as its temperature increases?**

The resistance also increases.

❑❑ **In a loop with a single battery and several resistors, in which direction will conventional current flow with respect to the battery terminals?**

From + to -

❑❑ **If one has a 6-V battery connected to three 2-Ω resistors in series, what is the potential drop across each resistor?**

The total current is 6V/6Ω=1A, so the potential drop across each resistor is $\Delta V = IR = (1A)(2\Omega) = 2$ V

❑❑ **If one has several resistors hooked up in parallel to a 6-V battery, what can be said about the potential drop across each resistor?**

The potential drop of resistors hooked in parallel is the same, so the potential drop across each resistor would be 6 V.

❑❑ **What is the effective resistance of a 6-Ω and 3-Ω resistor hooked in parallel?**

$R_{tot} = (3*6)/(3+6) = 18/9 = 2$ Ω

❑❑ **What is the difference between DC and AC?**

In DC (direct current), the current flows in one direction, while in AC (alternating current), the circuit oscillates its direction over time.

❑❑ **What is implied by the 60-hz frequency of a typical wall outlet?**

The voltage oscillates its polarity 60 times per second.

❑❑ **If an open RC circuit (a circuit with both resistance and capacitance) is closed (becomes conducting), what is the initial current, and how does it change over time?**

$I_o = \varepsilon/R$; as time goes on, the capacitor becomes charged and the voltage across it begins to approach the voltage of the battery. The current decays exponentially $I = I_o \exp(-t/RC)$.

MAGNETISM

❑❑　**What is the formula for the force experienced by a charge moving in a magnetic field (Lorentz's law)?**

F = q vxB (where 'x' implies a cross product, B = strength of the magnetic field [gauss], and q is a positive charge).

❑❑　**How does one find the direction of F in Lorentz's law, using the right hand rule?**

Fingers in direction of v, palm points in direction of B, thumb will point in direction of F.

❑❑　**How do the magnetic field lines run in a bar magnet?**

They exit the magnet from the "north" pole and enter the magnet at the "south" pole. Inside the magnet, they continue so that the magnetic field lines form loops.

❑❑　**Can a magnetic field speed up a moving charge?　Can it accelerate a moving charge?**

No - because the force is always directed perpendicular to the charge's velocity.　Yes - because the magnetic field changes the direction of the charge's velocity.

❑❑　**The current in a wire creates a magnetic field.　What can be said about the direction and magnitude of this field?**

The magnetic field runs in circles about the wire according to the right hand rule - point thumb in direction of current, and fingers will curl in the direction of the magnetic field. The magnetic field decreases as one gets farther away from the wire (B ∝ 1/r).

❑❑　**What are the units of magnetic field?**

Tesla (T) or Gauss (Ga);　10000 Gauss = 1 Tesla

❑ ❑ **What can one say about the polarity of the earth's magnetic field?**

Geographic north roughly coincides with the "magnetic south" of the earth's magnetic field. The magnetic north of a compass is attracted to this "magnetic south".

ELECTROMAGNETIC WAVES

❑❑ **What is the characteristic speed (c) of all electromagnetic (EM) waves in a vacuum?**

$c = 3.0 \times 10^8$ m/s.

❑❑ **How are the different EM waves arranged in order of increasing frequency (and energy per photon)?**

Radio waves, microwaves, infrared (IR), visible light (ROYBGV), ultraviolet (UV), x-ray, gamma ray.

❑❑ **What is the relation between wavelength and frequency for EM waves?**

$c = f\lambda$ where c = speed of light, f = frequency, and λ = wavelength.

❑❑ **What oscillates in an EM wave?**

An electric field oscillates perpendicular to the direction of propagation. Additionally, a magnetic field oscillates perpendicular to the direction of propagation and perpendicular to the electric field.

❑❑ **What occurs during polarization?**

A particular direction of the electric field oscillation is "selected" from the incoming light by some kind of filter.

OPTICS

❏❏ **What is the law of reflection in geometric optics?**

$\theta_{incident} = \theta_{reflected}$ where θ is the angle measured relative to the normal of the reflecting surface.

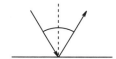

❏❏ **What does a material's index of refraction (n) signify, and how is it assigned?**

The index of refraction indicates how slowly light moves through the material. $n = c_{vacuum}/c_{material}$. Examples: $n_{air} \sim 1.0$, $n_{water} \sim 1.33$, $n_{glass} \sim 1.5$

❏❏ **What is Snell's law (law of refraction)?**

$n_1 \sin\theta_1 = n_2 \sin\theta_2$

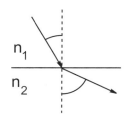

❏❏ **When incident light goes from a (slow) material with high n to a (fast) material with low n, what happens to the refracted beam?**

It is bent away from the normal.

❏❏ **Why does a prism break "white" light into its constituent colors?**

Because the index of refraction is different for different colors ($n_{violet} > n_{red}$), therefore some colors are "bent" more and separate into a continuous spectrum.

❏❏ **When does total internal reflection occur?**

When light traveling from a slow (high n) to a fast (low n) material approaches the boundary with a large angle ($\theta_1 > \theta_{critical}$) relative to the normal. (If one calculates θ_2 using Snell's law, there is no solution.)

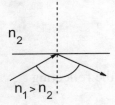

❏❏ **In a spherical mirror, how is the radius of curvature R related to the focal length f of the mirror?**

$f = R/2$

❏❏ **If an object is placed along a spherical mirror's central axis, a distance d_o from the mirror, how is image location d_i calculated?**

$1/f = 1/d_o + 1/d_i$

❏❏ **What is the difference between convex and concave mirrors?**

Convex mirrors (mirrored surface on the outside of the "bowl") have negative focal lengths ($f < 0$), and concave mirrors (mirrored surface on the inside of the "bowl") have positive focal lengths ($f > 0$). Convex mirrors can only form virtual images; concave mirrors can form both real and virtual images.

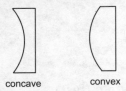

concave   convex

❏❏ **What is the difference between a real and a virtual image?**

A real image has light rays that actually pass through the image location (you could put a screen there and see the image). Virtual images only appear to be coming from the image location (e.g., your reflection in a bathroom mirror).

❏❏ **How does one interpret a negative image distance?**

The image is virtual.

❏❏ **How is magnification calculated?**

$M = h_i/h_o = -d_i/d_o$ (where h_i and h_o are the image and object heights, respectively).

❏❏ **What does a negative magnification (M<0) imply?**

The image is inverted.

❏❏ **If an object is placed along a lens's central axis, a distance d_o from the lens, how is image location d_i calculated?**

The same formula as is used for mirrors: $1/f = 1/d_o + 1/d_i$

❏❏ **How are converging and diverging lenses different?**

Converging lenses have positive focal lengths (f >0), while diverging lenses have negative focal lengths (f<0). Generally, converging lenses are thicker in the middle and thinner at the edges. The reverse is true for diverging lenses.

diverging   converging

❏❏ **What causes the interference pattern of Young's double slit experiment?**

The two slits serve as a source of expanding wavefronts that are in phase with each other. Bands of constructive and destructive interference show up as a series of light and dark bands on a screen.

❏❏ **What is a diffraction grating? What is the significance of a grating with 10000 lines/cm?**

A series of slits used to diffract light. The spacing between the slits would be 1 cm / $10000 = 1 \times 10^{-2}$ m/1 x $10^4 = 1 \times 10^{-6}$ m = 1000 nm.

❏❏ **What is the wavelength range of the visible light?**

About 400 nm (violet) to 700 nm (red).

❏❏ **What condition is required for diffraction of waves to occur through an opening?**

The size of the opening should be close to the wavelength.

❏❏ **What is an Angstrom?**

10^{-10} m (or 10 nm).

❏❏ **What is the formula for determining the location of bright spots resulting from a diffraction grating?**

$d\sin\theta = m\lambda$ where λ is the wavelength of light, d is the distance between lines on the grating, q is the angle between the incident beam and the mth order maxima (m=0,1,2, . . .)

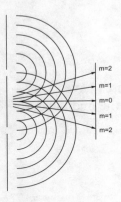

ATOMIC AND NUCLEAR PHYSICS

❏❏ **What is the energy (E) of a single photon?**

$E = hf$ where f is the frequency in Hz and h is Planck's constant.

❏❏ **In the photoelectric effect, how is the energy of incoming photons delivered to an electron?**

$hf = \phi + K$ where ϕ is the energy required to remove the electron from the material (also known as the work function), and K is the kinetic energy it has after leaving; if $hf < \phi$, the electron does not leave the material.

❏❏ **In the photoelectric effect experiment, why won't intense red light generate a current if the cutoff wavelength is in the green region?**

In order to eject an electron and generate a current, the photon must have a minimum amount of energy. The energy of a green photon is greater than that of a red photon. The latter does not deliver enough energy to overcome the work function of the metal.

❏❏ **In the hydrogen atom, the electron energy levels are "quantized". What does the spacing look like?**

As an electron moves up from the lowest energy (ground) state, the levels become increasingly close together. The energy of each level E_n varies as $E = -13.6 \text{ eV}/n^2$ (n = 1,2,...)

❏❏ **What photon energy would be required to excite an electron from n = 1 to n = 2 in a hydrogen atom?**

The energy of the photon would be the difference between the electron's initial energy E_1 and its final energy E_2. $E_{photon} = hf = \Delta E = E_2 - E_1 = -13.6 \text{ eV} (1/2^2 - 1/1^2) = -13.6 \text{ eV} (-3/4) \sim 10 \text{ eV}$

❏❏ **What is a half-life?**

The amount of time required for a given amount of radioactive material to decay to half its population.

❑❑ **Assume isotope A decays to isotope B with a half-life of 30 days. A sample that was originally pure A now has a B:A ratio of 7:1. How old is the sample? How old would you estimate the sample to be if the ratio was 10:1?**

The ratio of 7:1 implies that the remaining A isotope is 1/8 the original amount. The fraction is related to the number (n) of half-lives: $1/8 = (1/2)^n$ where n=3. The sample is 90 days old.

If the ratio is 10:1, then $1/11 = (1/2)^n$ and there is no easy solution. Since $(1/2)^3 = 1/8$ and $(1/2)^4 = 1/16$, the sample would be between 3 and 4 half-lives old (90-120 days).

❑❑ **What is an alpha (α) particle?**

A helium nucleus stripped of both electrons, $^4He2^+$ often emitted by heavy elements like U or Th.

❑❑ **What is a beta (β) particle?**

An electron (β^-) or positron (β^+) , often a decay product of a nucleus.

❑❑ **What is a gamma (γ) ray?**

A high-energy photon (hf >0.1 MeV), often released by an excited nucleus.

❑❑ **If the products of a nuclear reaction have less mass Δm than the original particles, has the law of mass conservation been violated?**

The law of conservation of mass-energy has not been violated. The mass Δm has been converted to energy $E = \Delta mc^2$.

❑❑ **What is the difference between fission and fusion?**

Fusion is the combining of two nuclei to form a larger nucleus. Fission is the breakup of a large nucleus into two or more particles.

AA **How do the original number (N_o) and activity (R_o) of radioactive particles change over time?**

nuclei = $N = N_o \exp(-\lambda t)$ activity (decays/s) = $R = R_o \exp(-\lambda t)$ where $t_{1/2} = \ln 2 /\lambda$.

❑❑ **If a ^{15}O nucleus undergoes β^+ decay, what nucleus is left (conservation of charge)?**

^{15}N

❑❑ **If an excited ^{39}K nucleus undergoes γ-decay, what nucleus is left?**

^{39}K. Gamma decay involves the emission of a high-energy photon, but no change in atomic number.

❑❑ **After $^{208}_{82}$Pb undergoes α-decay, how many protons and neutrons are left?**

Originally, Pb-208 has 82 protons and 208-82 = 126 neutrons. An α-particle removes 2 protons and 2 neutrons, leaving 80 protons and 124 neutrons.

❑❑ **How does one calculate the de Broglie wavelength of a particle from its momentum p?**

$\lambda = h / p$

BOTTOM LINE

This is a quick review. It is NOT intended to be complete and does not provide explanations or details. BUT, this is an excellent way to quickly review all major topics and points covered on the MCAT. All of the concepts reviewed here are discussed in more detail throughout this book. Good luck!

BIOLOGY BOTTOM LINE
CELLULAR RESPIRATION

$$C_6H_{12}O_6 + 6O_2 \rightarrow 6H_2O + 6CO_2 + Energy$$
(Glucose is oxidized to carbon dioxide)

	Substrate	Location	Type	Product
Glycolysis	**Glucose**	**Cytoplasm**	**Anaerobic and/or aerobic**	**2 ATP 2 NADH Pyruvate**
Krebs Cycle	**Acetyl CoA**	**Mitochondria (Eukaryotes) Plasma membrane (Prokaryotes)**	**Aerobic**	*** 1 GTP 3 NADH 1 FADH$_2$ 2 CO$_2$**
Electron Transport Chain	**NADH/FADH$_2$**	**Mitochondria (Eukaryotes) Plasma membrane (Prokaryotes)**	**Aerobic**	**ATP**

*Products per turn of Krebs cycle. One glucose molecule ultimately produces 2 pyruvates that form 2 acetyl-CoA and thus 2 turns of the cycle.

Facts:
- Glucose (6 carbons) is split to pyruvate (3 carbons) through glycolysis.
- If anaerobic (no oxygen), then pyruvate may be converted to lactic acid (NAD$^+$ is regenerated).
- If aerobic (oxygen present), then pyruvate is converted to acetyl-CoA and enters the Krebs cycle (and final products then enter the electron transport chain).
- In electron transport chain, NADH is converted to approximately 3 ATP, and FADH$_2$ is converted to approximately 2 ATP.
- Total net ATP from anaerobic respiration (i.e., glycolysis) is 2, whereas total net ATP generation from aerobic respiration is approximately 36.

Enzymes

❑   Biological *catalysts* that *speed* reaction.
❑   *Proteins* (almost exclusively).
❑   *No* effect on direction of reaction (speed BOTH forward and backward directions).
❑   *Not* consumed/changed in the reaction.

Negative Feedback

❑   A substance is produced which causes *inhibition* of substances that lead to its production. Thus, excess production of substance is prevented and control of production is attained.
❑   The majority of physiologic processes are controlled by this mechanism.
❑   Examples: hormone regulation, glycolysis.

Positive Feedback

❑   A substance is produced which causes *stimulation* of the substances that lead to its production. This in and of itself does NOT provide a mechanism to "turn off" the process or prevent excess.
❑   Examples: childbirth, action potential, ovulation.

MICROBIOLOGY

Viruses

- *Obligate intracellular parasites.*
- Do not have any of their own cellular machinery.
- Do not have membrane-bound organelles.
- Do have either RNA or DNA with protein core.

Bacteria

- *Prokaryotes* (No nucleus or membrane-bound organelles).
- Reproduce: *Binary Fission.*
- Pass genetic material through transposition, transformation, and conjugation.

Bacterial Shapes

Cocci	Spherical
Baccili	Rod-shaped
Spirochetes	Spiral

Gram Stain (for bacteria)

Positive: THICK layer of PEPTIDOGLYCAN in CELL WALL.
Negative: Very thin layer of peptidoglycan; has "outer membrane".
Penicillin inhibits formation of peptidoglycan and is best suited to kill **Gram positive** bacteria.

Fungi

- Yeasts (unicellular) and molds (multicellular).
- EUKARYOTES.
- Ergosterol instead of cholesterol in plasma membrane
  Chitin instead of peptidoglycan in cell wall.

Size

EUKARYOTES > *PROKARYOTES* > *VIRUSES*
(FUNGI) > **(BACTERIA)** > *VIRUSES*

CELLS

Membrane-bound organelles

Nucleus	**Contains DNA**
Nucleolus	**Ribosomes made here**
Endoplasmic Reticulum	**Membrane-bound network involved in transport of substances**
Smooth Endoplasmic Reticulum	**No ribosomes; involved in detoxification (such as in liver)**
Rough Endoplasmic Reticulum	**Have *ribosomes* Involved in protein synthesis**
Golgi Apparatus	**Packing/sorting of cellular products Cis face *receives* substances Trans face *releases* product**
Lysosomes	**Destroy/clean debris (pH = 5)**
Mitochondria	**Energy production (ATP)/ Site of aerobic respiration**

Plasma Membrane

- Selectively permeable
- **Phospholipid bilayer**: Hydro*philic* on *out*side
  Hydro*phobic* on *in*side
- Cholesterol for fluidity (keeps plasma membrane fluid during cold)

TRANSPORT

SIMPLE DIFFUSION	FACILITATED DIFFUSION	ACTIVE TRANSPORT
Down concentration gradient	Down concentration gradient using a *CARRIER PROTEIN*	May be against (usually) or with concentration gradient
No energy required	No energy required	*ENERGY* required
No saturation kinetics	Saturation kinetics	Saturation kinetics

Secondary Active Transport

One molecule (such as sodium) is *actively* pumped out of cell and creates a concentration gradient. The return of the molecule (e.g., sodium) is coupled with a *passive* co-transport of another molecule (e.g., glucose). Thus, glucose exhibits secondary active transport.

Osmosis

❑ Water flows from area of *lowest particle concentration to highest.*
❑ Depends on *TOTAL NUMBER* of particles, NOT the size of the particles.

Sodium-Potassium Pump

❑ Pumps 2 POTASSIUM **IN**TO cell.
❑ Pumps 3 SODIUM **OUT** of cell.
❑ *Active* Transport
  Memory tip: Think potass**IUN** (or potass**IN**) instead of potass**IUM**.
  Also: IN (two letters) and OUT (three letters).

Sodium

❑ Predominant *extracellular* cation.

❑ Rushes into cell to initiate action potential.

Potassium

❑ Predominant *intracellular* cation.

❑ Rushes out of cell to re-polarize membrane.

Calcium

❑ Rushes into synaptic knob to cause binding of vesicles to synaptic membrane (which then release neurotransmitter into the synaptic cleft).

❑ Released from sarcoplasmic reticulum to cause *muscle contraction*
   - causes increased heart contraction (by contraction of cardiac muscle).
   - causes vasoconstriction (by contraction of smooth muscle).
   - causes movement (by contraction of skeletal muscle).

NERVOUS SYSTEM

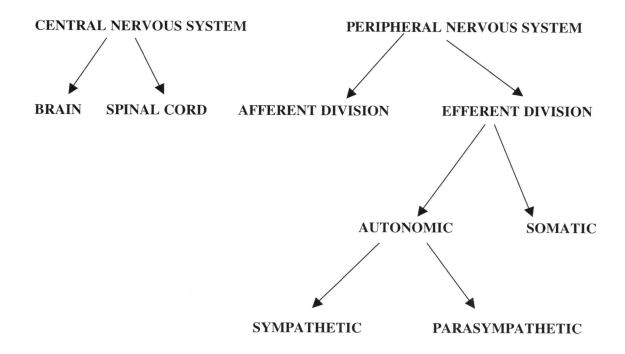

PERIPHERAL NERVOUS SYSTEM

AFFERENT	EFFERENT
Sensory	**Motor**
One neuron **(from periphery to CNS)**	**One or two neurons** **(from CNS to periphery)**
Dorsal root entrance	**Ventral root exit**
Dorsal root ganglion **(cell bodies are in)**	**Ventral horn** **(cell bodies are in)**
NO dendrites (have receptor cells)	**Have dendrites**
Mostly OUTSIDE CNS **(cell body, most of axon, receptor)**	**Mostly INSIDE CNS** **(cell body, dendrites, part of axon)**

<u>Memory Tip</u>: "**E**" for exit; **E**fferents "exit the spinal cord".
<u>Memory Tip #2</u>: "**V**" is part of an "**M**". Therefore, **v**entral is associated with **m**otor.

EFFERENT NERVOUS SYSTEM

SOMATIC	AUTONOMIC
Generally voluntary	Generally involuntary
SKELETAL muscle	*SMOOTH* muscle, *CARDIAC* muscle, and *GLANDS*
Leads to muscle excitation only	Can excite (EPSP) or inhibit (IPSP)
One neuron (acetylcholine)	Two-neuron relay
No further divisions	Sympathetic and Parasympathetic

Action potential (AP)
- Set off when a threshold potential is reached (usually –50 mEV).
- An action potential is *ALL or NONE*.
- Sodium ion RUSHES INTO axon causing depolarization.
- Has a refractory period before another AP can occur.

AP rushes down length of neuron to synaptic knob where:
- Calcium channels open and *calcium rushes into synaptic knob.*
- Vesicles with neurotransmitters release contents into synaptic cleft by exocytosis.

Neurotransmitters
- Travel in *ONE DIRECTION*…from synaptic knob to adjacent cell/muscle.
- They bind receptor cells and cause:
  1- Depolarization (excitatory) for muscle contraction (*Somatic* nervous system)
  2- EPSP or IPSP (*Autonomic* nervous system)
- *Acetylcholine* is used in all peripheral synaptic junctions except the second synaptic junction of the sympathetic nervous system.
- *Acetylcholinesterase* is an enzyme which breaks down acetylcholine (can be inhibited by certain medications and/or poisons).

AUTONOMIC NERVOUS SYSTEM

SYMPATHETIC	PARASYMPATHETIC
Fight or flight	Rest and digest
Relay in sympathetic chain	Relay on or close to target organ
Smooth muscle, cardiac muscle, or glands	Smooth muscle, cardiac muscle, or glands
Acetylcholine then norepinephrine	Acetylcholine then acetylcholine
Increased heart rate Dilated pupils Increased diameter of bronchioles Constriction of blood vessels Glycolysis Sweating	Decreased heart rate Constricted pupils Decreased diameter of bronchioles No innervation of blood vessels Digestion (increased peristalsis)

RESPIRATORY SYSTEM

Functions

❑ Gas exchange.
❑ Thermoregulation (questionable if occurs but is listed in MCAT student manual).
❑ Protection against disease (mucociliary pump).

Gas Exchange

❑ Occurs via *simple diffusion* at capillary-alveoli border.

Oxygen-Hemoglobin Curve (UNDERSTAND concept behind this!!!!)

❑ Shifts to right: High CO_2, low pH, increased temperature.
❑ Shifts to left: Low CO_2, high pH, lower temperature, CO poisoning.
❑ Shift to right → p50 increases (more oxygen RELEASED to tissues).
❑ Shift to left → p50 decreases (less oxygen released to tissues).

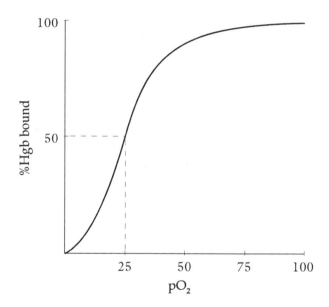

CIRCULATORY SYSTEM

Functions

- Transport oxygen to tissues; remove carbon dioxide from tissues
- Transport nutrients
- Immune system
- Thermoregulation

Pulmonary Circulation

Right Atrium → Right Ventricle → Pulmonary Artery → Lungs → left atrium

Systemic Circulation

Left Atrium → Left Ventricle → Aorta → Body (tissues) → right atrium

Vasculature

Arteries: Away from heart
Vein: Toward the heart
Artery → Arterioles → Capillaries → Venules → Veins

Systole: *Contraction* phase of heart

Diastole: *Relaxation* phase of heart

Blood pressure = systolic/diastolic

Blood Composition

1- Plasma (55%)
2- Cells (45%) includes:
   Red blood cells (erythrocytes): carry *oxygen* to tissues; help transport carbon dioxide to lungs.
   White blood cells (leukocytes): involved in *immune* system; increase in number during infection.
   Platelets (thrombocytes): involved with blood clotting.

IMMUNE SYSTEM

Antigen: Foreign body

Cell Mediated Immunity
- T-lymphocytes
- Best for viruses, fungi, intracellular bacteria
- Helper T cells (mediate), cytotoxic T cells (attack), suppressor T cells (shut down)
- HIV attacks helper T cells.

Humoral Immunity
- B-lymphocytes
- Best for extracellular bacteria
- B lymphocytes → plasma cells → antibodies.

Complement
- "Complements" humoral and cell-mediated immune system
- Forms attack membrane complex which attacks cells marked by antibodies.

ALL blood cells originate in ***BONE MARROW***.
B-lymphocytes MATURE in *B*one marrow.
T-lymphocytes MATURE in *T*hymus.

DIGESTION

Oral Cavity
- *Polysaccharide* digestion begins by salivary amylase
- Food forms bolus

Esophagus
- *Transport* of food only

Stomach
- HCl secreted from parietal cells causing acid environment (pH about 2).
- Acid destroys salivary amylase (NO polysaccharide digestion).
- Acid converts pepsinogen (from chief cells) to pepsin.
- *PROTEIN* digestion begins with acid and pepsin.

Small Intestine
- Sodium bicarbonate neutralizes acid and pH increases.
- *LARGEST SURFACE AREA* (*most of digestion* takes place here).
- Carbohydrate and protein digestion occur with use of pancreatic enzymes (see pancreas).
- Fat digestion is aided by emulsification with bile produced in liver and occurs via lipase produced in pancreas.
- *Carbohydrate/proteins* -> Taken up into *capillary* system and eventually to liver.
- *Fat* -> Taken up into the *lymphatic* system by *lacteals* in the villi.

Large Intestine
- Some residual digestion but mostly *stool formation* via reabsorbtion of sodium and water.

Liver
- *Produces bile*
- Detoxification

Gallbladder
- *STORES bile*
- Secreted with meals to emulsify fats

Pancreas

Exocrine functions:

- ❑ Carbohydrate digestion: produces amylase
- ❑ Protein digestion: produces trypsin, chymotrypsin, and carboxypeptidase
- ❑ Fat digestion: produces lipase

Endocrine functions:

- ❑ Glucagon – stimulates glucose formation from glycogen (storage form)
- ❑ Insulin – allows for glucose uptake into cells (excreted after eating)
- ❑ Somatostatin

Exocrine versus Endocrine

An ***exo***crine gland secretes substance into ***ducts***, whereas ***endo***crine means secretion of substance into the ***bloodstream***. The pancreas has both exocrine and endocrine functions.

MUSCLE

Type of muscle	Skeletal	Smooth	Cardiac
Structure	Striations	No striations	Striations and intercalated discs
Nervous system innervation	Somatic	Autonomic	Myogenic with autonomic modification
Voluntary or involuntary	Generally voluntary	Generally involuntary	Generally involuntary
Location	Attached to bones of both axial and appendicular skeleton	Digestive tract, reproductive tract, vasculature (mostly arteries/arterioles)	Heart
Components	Troponin/ tropomyosin	No troponin	Troponin/ tropomyosin

Skeletal muscle contraction
- CALCIUM is released from the *SARCOPLASMIC RETICULUM*. Next the calcium binds with TROPONIN which then pulls TROPOMYOSIN out of the way and allows for the attachment of ACTIN and MYOSIN. The linkage of actin and myosin requires energy (ATP).

Remember: In general, skeletal muscle contraction is fast and strong, whereas smooth muscle contraction is slower and weaker but is long-lasting.

Tendons
- Attach *muscle to bone.*

Ligaments
- Attach *bone to bone*

Bone

- OsteoBlasts: **B**uild bone ("**B**LASTS **B**UILD")
- OsteoClasts: resorbs (breaks down bone... "**C**LASTS **C**OLLAPSE")
- Osteocytes: bone cells
- Parathryroid hormone: stimulates osteoclasts → increases blood Ca^{++}
- Calcitonin: inhibits osteoclasts → decrease blood Ca^{++}

Skin (functions)

- Homeostasis
- Osmoregulation
- Thermoregulation
  Vasodilation: loss of heat
  Vasoconstriction: conserve heat
- Physical protection

Kidney

- *Regulates sodium/water balance*
- Regulates blood pressure (renin-angiotensin-aldosterone system)
- Stimulates RBC production (erythropoietin)
- Concentrate/dilute urine

REPRODUCTION

Prokaryotes: Binary fission
Eukaryotes: Mitosis, Meiosis

Mitosis vs. Meiosis

Mitosis

- ONE division (prophase, metaphase, anaphase, telophase)
- Produces TWO diploid daughter cells IDENTICAL to mother cell.

Meiosis

- TWO divisions (prophase, metaphase, anaphase, telophase) without interphase (DNA replication) in between
- Produces FOUR haploid daughter cells NOT identical to mother cell.

Cell Cycle

1-Interphase (metabolic and DNA replication)
2-Division of chromosomes (mitosis/meiosis)
3-Division of cytoplasm (cytokinesis)

Spermatogenesis

- Spermatogonia -> spermatogonia (mitosis)
- Spermatogonia -> spermatids (meiosis)
- Stimulated by FSH
- Takes place in SEMINIFEROUS TUBULES.

Oogenesis

- Born with total number of oogonia
- Oogonium -> Ovum over extended time period
- Unequal amount of cytoplasm dispensed (polar bodies form)
- Maturation of follicle: FSH
- Ovulation: LH

Fertilization takes place in FALLOPIAN TUBES (OVIDUCT) and the zygote travels to the uterus for implantation. Mitotic division then takes place to form a multicellular organism.

CELL DIFFERENTIATION

Endoderm	Mesoderm	Ectoderm
Thyroid Bladder Liver Pancreas Lungs Lining of some internal organs	Bone Muscle Blood cells Kidneys Gonads	Hair Nails Epidermis Lens of the eye Nervous system Epithelium of the nose, mouth, and anus

GENERAL CHEMISTRY BOTTOM LINE

THE BASICS

Sub-atomic Particles

	CHARGE	LOCATION	MASS
PROTON	+1	In nucleus	Equal to neutron
ELECTRON	-1	Surrounds nucleus	1/1800 of n.or p.
NEUTRON	0	In nucleus	Equal to proton

Empirical vs. Molecular Formula

Empirical formula	Smallest ratio of whole numbers (e.g., CH)
Molecular formula	Actual chemical composition (e.g., C_5H_5)

Mole Concept

1 Mole = 6.02×10^{23} atoms
(based on number of atoms in 12 grams of carbon)

Oxidation/Reduction Reactions

Oxidation	Loses electrons (becomes more positive)
Reduction	Gains electrons (becomes more negative)
Oxidizing agent	Oxidizes *substance* that it reacts with, but the oxidizing agent itself is reduced
Reducing agent	Reduces *substance* that it reacts with, but the reducing agent itself becomes oxidized

PERIODIC TABLE TRENDS

Period (horizontal) [as you go from *left to right*]
- Atomic radius decreases
- Ionization energy increases
- Electronegativity increases
- Electron affinity increases

Group (vertical) [as you go *down* the group]
- Atomic radius increases
- Ionization energy decreases
- Electronegativity decreases
- Electron affinity decreases

Atomic Number: number of protons

Mass Number: protons + neutrons

Formal Charge
(Atomic number) – (# of bonds) – (# of lone pair electrons)

Density
Density = Mass/Volume (D=M/V)

Density = (P)(MM)/(R)(T) where P = pressure, MM = molar mass, R = constant, T = temperature

Kinetic Energy
$KE = \frac{1}{2} mv^2$

BONDING

Ionic bonding	*Transfer* of electrons	Between a *metal* and a *non-metal*	Example: NaCl
Covalent bonding	*Sharing* of electrons	Between two *non-metals*	Example: HCl

Partial Ionic Character

Remember that not all bonding is completely ionic or completely covalent. Thus, many bonds have characteristics of both.

Hydrogen Bonding

❑ *Intermolecular* attraction between partial positive hydrogen and partial negative molecule
❑ Highly electronegative molecule must be fluorine, oxygen, or nitrogen.

Memory tip: Hydrogen is a "FON" bond: F-fluorine, O-oxygen, N-nitrogen.

Van der Waals Forces

❑ Intermolecular forces formed by weak interactions (attractive and repulsive forces) between molecules
❑ Very weak forces

Bond Strength

Covalent > ionic > hydrogen > van der Waals

Bond Dissociation Energy

❑ Enthalpy per mole required to break one type of bond in a molecule

Safety Tip: *Energy is needed to break bonds*, whereas *energy is given off when bonds are formed*. This simple statement is often confused. Thus, take a moment to understand as well as memorize this.

ACID AND BASE CHEMISTRY

Type	Arrhenius	Bronsted-Lowry	Lewis
ACID	Forms *hydronium* (H_3O^+) in aqueous solution	Donates hydrogen	Accepts electrons
BASE	Forms *hydroxide* (OH^-) in aqueous solution	Accepts hydrogen	Donates electrons

Note: An Arrhenius acid is by definition a Bronsted acid and a Lewis acid.
BUT, a Lewis acid is not necessarily a Bronsted or Arrhenius acid (e.g., hydrogen may not be involved).

$pH = -\log [H^+]$
$pOH = -\log [OH^-]$
$pK_a = -\log [K_a]$
$pK_b = -\log [K_b]$

Ionization of Water

$K_w = [H^+] [OH^-] = 10^{-14}$ at STP
Thus, $p[H^+] + p[OH] = 14$
And, $K_w = K_a K_b$

Strong Acids

- HCl, H_2SO_4, HI, HNO_3, HBr, $HClO_4$
- Completely dissociate in solution

Strong Bases

- $NaOH$, $LiOH$, KOH
- Completely dissociate in solution

Weak Acids and Weak Bases

- Only partially dissociate in solution
- Form good buffers

BUFFERS

Characteristics of a Good Buffer

- $pH = pK_a$ (the closer the pK_a is to the pH, the better the buffer)
- Large amount of weak acid/weak base

Henderson-Hasselbalch Equation

$pH = pK_a + log$ [base/acid]

When *conjugate base = conjugate acid,* then *$pH=pK_a$.* This is the point where the buffer works best. Note that this is *not* the equivalence point.

Equivalence point (pI): Point at which total chemical base = total chemical acid.

Safety Tip: Remember that this formula can be written in slightly different forms such as $pK_a = pH - log$ [base/acid]. Memorize one form, but be able to recognize other correct and incorrect forms on the MCAT (via simple algebra).

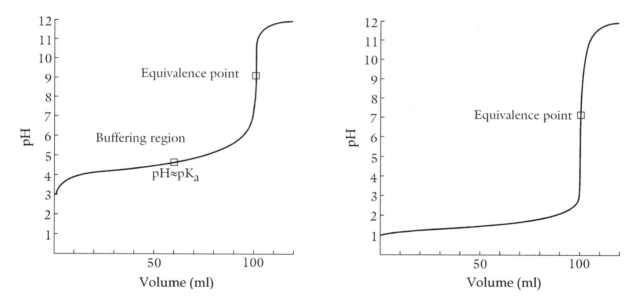

The graph on the left represents a titration of a weak acid with a weak base. The graph on the right represents the titration of a strong acid with a strong base. Contrast the starting pHs of the two graphs as well as the shape of the curves.

THERMODYNAMICS

Enthalpy: Measure of heat content (H); at constant pressure, the amount of heat absorbed by a substance is equal to change in enthalpy (ΔH).

Exothermic	$-\Delta H$	Heat energy released during reaction
Endothermic	$+\Delta H$	Heat energy put into reaction

Entropy: Measure of disorder (S)

ΔS universe = ΔS surroundings + ΔS system
(entropy of the universe is always increasing [2nd Law of Thermodynamics])

$\Delta S = \Delta S$ products - ΔS reactants

Increased disorder: $+\Delta S$
Decreased disorder: $^-\Delta S$

Gibbs Free Energy: Measure of free energy (G)

$\Delta G = \Delta H - T\,\Delta S$

If $\Delta G > 0$, reaction is *non-spontaneous.*
If $\Delta G = 0$, reaction is *equilibrium.*
If $\Delta G < 0$, reaction is *spontaneous.*

Enthalpy (ΔH)	Entropy (ΔS)	Gibbs Free Energy (ΔG)	? Spontaneous
+	-	+	No
-	+	-	Yes
+	+	+/-	At high temperatures
-	-	+/-	At low temperatures

EQUILIBRIUM

$2A + B \leftrightarrow C + D$

$$K = \frac{[C][D]}{[A]^2[B]}$$

K > 1 → Products > reactants → reaction is "toward the right"
K < 1 → Reactants > products → reaction is "toward the left"
K = 1 → Products = reactants → equilibrium

Remember:

- Liquids and solids do **not** factor into the equilibrium expression…only aqueous solutions and gases are used to calculate this.
- The molar coefficient such as "2A" becomes $[A]^2$ in the equilibrium equation.
- K is constant for a given reaction as long as temperature is held constant.

Relationship between ΔG and K

$\Delta G = \text{-RT lnK}$

When $\Delta G > 0$ → K<1 → reactants > products → non-spontaneous
When $\Delta G = 0$ → K=1 → reactants = products → equilibrium
When $\Delta G < 0$ → K>1 → products > reactants → spontaneous

LeChatelier's Principle

Definition: If a stress is applied to a system at equilibrium, the system will shift in the direction that minimizes the effects of that stress.

Increase in pressure shifts the reaction *toward the side* with the *fewer total moles of gas.*
Increase in temperature shifts the reaction *away from the side that contains heat* in the equation (i.e., toward the left in exothermic reactions and toward the right in endothermic reactions.
Removing a substance shifts the reaction *toward the side of removal.*
Adding a substance shifts the reaction *away from the side of addition.*
Adding or removing a *catalyst* does *not* shift the direction of the reaction.

KINETICS

Reaction rate is determined **EXPERIMENTALLY**. On the MCAT you may be given the results of an experiment and expected to determine the reaction order (see examples in body of this book or in practice MCATs). Another possibility is that you are given an elementary step of a reaction. In other words, you are given one step of the series of steps which make up a reaction. In this case you *can* determine the reaction order. If this information is not given, you cannot determine the reaction rate.

$A + B \longleftrightarrow C + D$

$\text{rate} = k\,[A]^x[B]^y$

X= the coefficient of A
Y= the coefficient of B

Rate Law
- Dependent on concentration of *reactants*
- Determined *experimentally*
- The order of the reaction can be found by adding exponents or superscripts (x + y in above example) in an *experimentally determined* rate law.

GASES

Ideal Gas
- ❑ Occupy no volume
- ❑ Constant state of random motion
- ❑ Exert no forces on each other
- ❑ Collisions are elastic (no loss of energy from friction).

Real Gases
- ❑ In reality, gases do not hold all of the properties of an "ideal" gas. Forces *do* exist between gas particles. These forces are termed *van der Waals forces*. These repulsive forces increase when *temperature is low* and *pressure is high*.

Ideal gas law: $PV = nRT$ (Memorize this and all others can be derived from it.)

Avogadro's Law: $V_1/n_1 = V_2/n_2$
Boyle's Law: $P_1V_1 = P_2V_2$
Charles' Law: $V_1/T_1 = V_2/T_2$
P=pressure, V=volume, n=number of moles, R=gas constant, T=temperature

Standard Temperature and Pressure (STP)
P = 1 atm (760 mmHg or 760 torr), T = 0° C (273 K)
1 Mole of gas at STP = 22.4 liters

Dalton's Law of Partial Pressures
(Partial pressure of X) = (Total pressure) (Mole fraction of X)

Mole fraction = mole of X/total moles

Graham's Law of Effusion
The ratio of the effusion rate of two gases is inversely proportional to the square root of the ratio of their molecular weights:

$R_1/R_2 = [M_2/M_1]^{1/2}$ R=gas, M=molecular weight

SOLUTION CHEMISTRY

Molarity: number of moles per liter of solution.

Molality: number of moles per kilogram of solvent.

Normality: number of equivalents of either acid or base (e.g., H_2SO_4 -> Norm = 2).

Triple point: the point at which the three phases of matter co-exist in equilibrium.

Solution: a homogenous system that contains two or more substances.

Miscible solution: two solutions that when mixed together form a one-phase solution.

Immiscible solution: two solutions that form a two-phase solution when mixed.

Colligative Properties (property of a solution based on the number of solute particles without regard to the particular identity of the solution)

1-Vapor pressure lowering
2-Freezing point depression
3-Boiling point elevation
4-Osmotic pressure

ELECTROCHEMISTRY

Reduction takes place at the cathode, whereas oxidation takes place at the anode. When combining two half-cells, reduction takes place at the cell with *the more positive charge.*

Standard half-cell reduction potential (ΔE^{o}): $E^{o} = E^{o}$ (cathode) $- E^{o}$ (anode)

Relationship between ΔG and E^{o}: $\Delta G^{o} = -nFE^{o}$

Memory Tip: Think *RED CAT* (i.e., reduction takes place at the cathode)

Galvanic cell: two half-cell substances react *spontaneously.*

Electrolytic cell: the reaction is *non-spontaneous* and requires the input of electricity in order to propel the reaction.

ORGANIC CHEMISTRY BOTTOM LINE

NOMENCLATURE

PREFIX	# OF CARBONS
METH-	1
ETH-	2
PROP-	3
BUT-	4
PENT-	5
HEX-	6
HEPT-	7
OCT-	8
NON-	9
DEC-	10

Suffixes (from highest to lowest priority):

• **Carboxylic acids (-oate) and derivatives**
• **Aldehydes (-al)**
• **Ketones (-one)**
• **Alcohols (-ol)**
• **Amines (-amine)**
• **Alkynes (-yne)**
• **Alkenes (-ene)**
• **Alkanes (-ane)**

1- Find the *longest chain* -> name it.
   Prefix: Number of carbons in a chain determines this (as noted above).
   Suffix: Derived after determining the functional group involved. If more than one functional group is noted, the "highest priority" group should be determined.
2- Number the chain starting from end closest to functional group.
3- Identify any substituents and their locations (1-methyl, 2-methyl, etc.)
4- If more than one of the same substituent, then use di- (two), tri- (three), tetra- (four), etc.
5- List alphabetically without regard to di, tri, tetra, etc.

BONDING

Covalent: Sharing of electrons (two non-metals)

Ionic: Transfer of electrons (metal and non-metal)

Hydrogen: Intermolecular bond between hydrogen from $^-$OH to lone pair electrons of Fluorine, Oxygen, or Nitrogen ("FON" "bon"d)

	sp^3	sp^2	sp^1
Geometry	Tetrahedral	Planar	Linear
Angle (°)	109°	120°	180°
Bonds or lone pair electrons	4	3	2
Type of bonds	4 sigma bonds	3 sigma, 1 pi bond	2 sigma, 2 pi bonds

Multiple bonding (i.e., double bond, triple bond)

❑ Increased number of bonds, *decreases the length* of the bond.
❑ Increased number of bonds, *increases the energy* in the bond.

Bond formation/breaking bonds

❑ Energy is *needed to break* bonds (endothermic).
❑ Energy is *given off* when bonds are *formed* (exothermic).

Boiling Point

❑ The *longer* the carbon chain, the *higher* the boiling point.
❑ The *more branching* of equal-length carbon chains, the *lower* the boiling point.
    <u>Safety tip</u>: Boiling point deals with *intermolecular*, not intramolecular, forces.

ALKANES

Characteristics:

- Saturated hydrocarbon
- General formula: C_nH_{2n+2}
- Inert with most substances
- sp^3 hybridization of carbon

Reactions:

1. Combustion:

$$CH_4 + 2O_2 \rightarrow CO_2 + H_2O + Energy$$

Heat of combustion is the heat energy given off during the combustion reaction. The *higher the heat of combustion*, the *less stable* the carbon compound that was reacted.

2. Halogenation:

$$R\text{-}H + Cl_2 \xrightarrow{\text{light}} R\text{-}Cl + HCl$$

Mechanism: Free radical reaction ($3° > 2° > 1°$)
               Light is catalyst

Initiation:	$Cl\text{-}Cl \xrightarrow{\text{light}} 2Cl\bullet$
Propagation:	$R\text{-}H + Cl\bullet \longrightarrow R\bullet + HCl$
	$R\bullet + Cl_2 \longrightarrow R\text{-}Cl + Cl\bullet$
Termination:	$R\bullet + R\bullet \longrightarrow R\text{-}R$
	$R\bullet + Cl\bullet \longrightarrow R\text{-}Cl$
	$Cl\bullet + Cl\bullet \longrightarrow Cl\text{-}Cl$

Hydrocarbons: molecules with hydrogen (hence, "hydro") and carbon

Saturated hydrocarbon: "saturated" with hydrogens (single bonds)

Unsaturated hydrocarbon: not fully saturated with hydrogen (double and/or triple bonds)

ALKENES

Characteristics:

- Unsaturated hydrocarbons that contain one or more double bonds
- General formula: C_nH_{2n}
- Double bond (sigma bond of sp^2 hybridization + pi bond)

Reactions:

1. Electrophilic addition:
    - Electrophile: "Electron-loving." An electrophile attacks electrons.
    - Markovnikov: hydrogen adds to the side with the least carbon substitutions
    - Anti-Markovnikov: opposite of Markovnikov
    - Syn: Add to the same side of the double bond
    - Anti: Add to opposite side of the double bond
    - Random: May add to either side of the double bond

Markovnikov/ Random

Anti

Anti-Markovnikov/ Random

Markovnikov/ Anti

2. Reduction:
   - Addition of hydrogens
   - Add in syn position (both hydrogens add on the same side)
   - Reduction with $NaBH_4$ and $LiAlH_4$ does NOT occur with alkenes

Heterogeneous catalyst: catalyst is *different* chemical state than other reactants.

Homogeneous catalyst: catalyst is *same* chemical state as other reactants.

3. Oxidative Cleavage

Safety Tip: $KMnO_4/H_2O$ is another popular choice for oxidative cleavage.

ALKYNES

Characteristics:

- Unsaturated hydrocarbons that contain a triple bond
- General formula: C_nH_n
- Triple bond (sigma bond of sp^1 hybridization + 2 pi bonds)

Reactions:

1. Electrophilic addition
2. Reductions
3. Oxidations

Same reactions that occur with alkenes

ALCOHOLS

Characteristics:

- ❑ Hydrocarbons with hydroxyl group
- ❑ Can form intermolecular hydrogen bonds (⁻OH group)
- ❑ In general, soluble with <5 carbon chain
- ❑ Polar and protic (can be used as solvents or nucleophiles for S_N1 reactions)
- ❑ sp^3 hybridized oxygen

Reactions:

1. Elimination (E1): see section on elimination
2. Substitution: (S_N2 and S_N1)
   A) S_N1 reactions (on $2°$ or $3°$) often seen with *ethanol and heat*
   B) S_N2 reactions will occur on primary alcohol that is protonated (PBr_3 or $SOCl_2$ create better leaving group)
3. Oxidation

S_N2 reaction:

$$CH_3CH_2\text{-}OH \xrightarrow{PBr_3} \xrightarrow{HBr} CH_3CH\text{-}Br \quad + \quad HOPBr_2$$

S_N1 reaction:

Oxidation reactions:

NUCLEOPHILIC SUBSTITUTION REACTIONS

S_N1 (S = substitution, N = nucleophilic, 1= first order)
S_N2 (S = substitution, N = nucleophilic, 2 = second order)

	S_N1	S_N2
Reaction order	First-order reaction Rate=k [substrate]	Second-order reaction Rate=k [substrate] [Nu]
Mechanism	Carbocation	Backside attack
Stability order	$3^\circ > 2^\circ > 1^\circ$	$1^\circ > 2^\circ$
Products (if chiral)	Racemic	Inverted configuration
Rearrangements?	Yes (because of carbocation)	No
Favorable solvent	Polar protic	Polar aprotic

Examples of S_N1/S_N2 reactions

$$\underset{\underset{\displaystyle CH_3}{|}}{\overset{\overset{\displaystyle CH_3}{|}}{H_3C-C-OH}} \quad \xrightarrow{HBr} \quad \underset{\underset{\displaystyle CH_3}{|}}{\overset{\overset{\displaystyle CH_3}{|}}{H_3C-C\oplus}} \quad \xrightarrow{Br-} \quad \underset{\underset{\displaystyle CH_3}{|}}{\overset{\overset{\displaystyle CH_3}{|}}{H_3C-C-Br}}$$

Example of S_N1 reaction: Note the tertiary carbon and the carbocation intermediate.

$$\underset{\underset{\displaystyle H}{|}}{\overset{\overset{\displaystyle H}{|}}{H_3C-C-OH}} \quad \xrightarrow{HBr} \quad \underset{\underset{\displaystyle H}{|}}{\overset{\overset{\displaystyle H}{|}}{H_3C-C-OH}} \quad \longrightarrow \quad \underset{\underset{\displaystyle H}{|}}{\overset{\overset{\displaystyle H}{|}}{H_3C-C-Br}}$$

Example of an S_N2 reaction: Note the primary carbon and the lack of a carbocation intermediate. Instead, the reaction takes place by a "backside attack."

$$\underset{\underset{\displaystyle H}{|}}{\overset{\overset{\displaystyle H}{|}}{H_3C-C-OH}} \quad \xrightarrow{CH_3CH_2OH} \quad \text{NO REACTION}$$

This reaction (or rather LACK of reaction) illustrates the point that –OH is a bad leaving group. Note that the two previous reactions were able to proceed because the –OH was protonated by HBr.

Leaving Groups

- In general, *weaker bases* make *better* leaving groups.
- Decreasing reactivity: ***Tosylate- > I- > Br- > Cl- = H₂O***
- Safety tip: ⁻OH is a *bad* leaving group. If ⁻OH is protonated by an acid and becomes H_2O, then it is a *good* leaving group. But remember that ⁻OH *must* receive a H⁺ first!

Nucleophiles

Examples: H:⁻, CN:⁻, :SH⁻, ⁻:OH, ⁻:NH₂
Strength of nucleophiles: (follows some general trends)
1. Usually *increases going down column* in periodic table.
    Example: HS⁻ is better nucleophile than HO⁻
    I⁻ > Br⁻ > Cl⁻
2. Nucleophilicity roughly parallels basicity; the *more basic -> the better nucleophile*.

Rearrangements

Hydrogen shift

Note: Same principle applies for rearrangements with methyl group (i.e., methyl shift).

ELIMINATION

	E1	E2
Reaction order	First-order reaction	Second-order reaction
Stability order	$3^o > 2^o$	$3^o > 2^o > 1^o$
Product	Double bond (most highly substituted alkene)	Double bond
Geometry	Random	ANTI geometry

Remember: E1 typically occurs in conjunction with S_N1 and never occurs on a 1° carbon. E2 is most favored on a 3° carbon and needs only base to react when this is the case. In the case of a primary carbon, E2 will occur only if a very strong base such as tert-butyoxide is present.

ETHERS

$$CH_3\text{-}CH_2\text{-}O\text{-}CH_2\text{-}CH_3 \quad + \quad HBr \quad \rightarrow \quad CH_3\text{-}CH_2\text{-}OH \quad + \quad CH_3\text{-}CH_2\text{-}Br$$

- *Inert* with most substances
- *Do react with acids* as noted above (Usually S_N2 as noted in above reaction, but can be S_N1 if tertiary, allylic, or benzylic carbon is involved)
- sp^3 hybridized oxygen orbital

EPOXIDES

Characteristics:
- Subset of ethers (still considered ether!)
- Three member ring (two carbons and one oxygen)
- Highly strained because of bond angles

Reaction:
Nucleophilic substitution of carbon

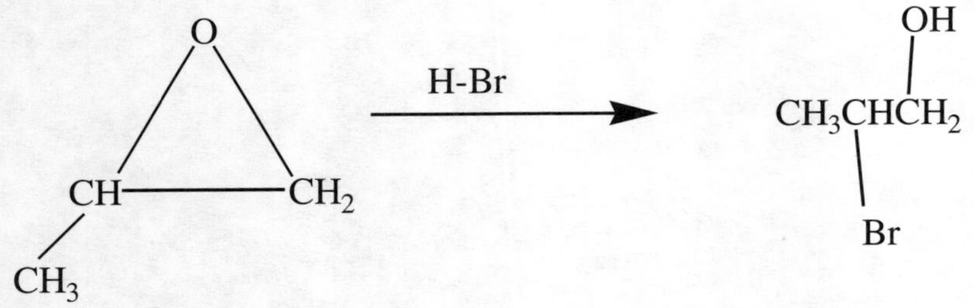

ALDEHYDES AND KETONES

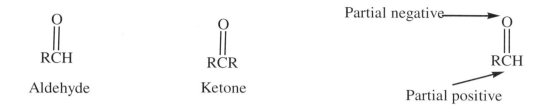

Aldehyde

Ketone

Partial negative →

Partial positive →

Facts:

- ❑ Aldehydes react faster than ketones.
- ❑ Aldehydes are less stable than ketones.
- ❑ Aldehydes/ketones have higher boiling points than equivalent hydrocarbons.
- ❑ Aldehydes/ketones have lower boiling points than equivalent alcohols.

Reactions:

1. Reduction:

$$CH_3CH \xrightarrow{\text{NaBH}_4} CH_3CH_2$$

Common reducing agents: $NaBH_4$, $LiAlBH_4$ (have negative hydrogen)

2. Oxidation:

$$CH_3CH \xrightarrow[\text{NH}_4\text{OH, H}_2\text{O}]{\text{Ag}_2\text{O}} CH_3COH$$

Common oxidizing agents: CrO_3, $KMnO_4$

3. Nucleophilic addition:

$$CH_3CH \xrightarrow{\text{HCN}} CH_3C\text{---CN}$$

4. Aldol condensation:

Acid or Base Catalyst

May undergo further dehydration
depending on reaction conditions

5. Acetal/ketal/hemiacetal/hemiketal formation:

Note: The acetal serves as a good "protecting group." That is, since the acetal is inert to
most substances, this "protects" the compound from undergoing unwanted reactions. An
acetal can be reversed with acid as follows.

Trick for deriving products for reverse acetal reaction:
1. Find the point of attachment (the carbon that the two oxygens attach to).
2. Eliminate the bond between the oxygen molecules and the carbon.
3. Add hydrogen to the oxygen molecules.
4. Add a double-bonded oxygen to the "point of attachment" carbon.

Example:

BENZENE

Characteristics:

❑ Aromatic
❑ Electrophilic addition and nucleophilic substitution (under certain conditions such as strong base) may occur, but otherwise benzene is inert to most substances.

Reactions:

1. Electrophilic substitution (E = Electrophile)

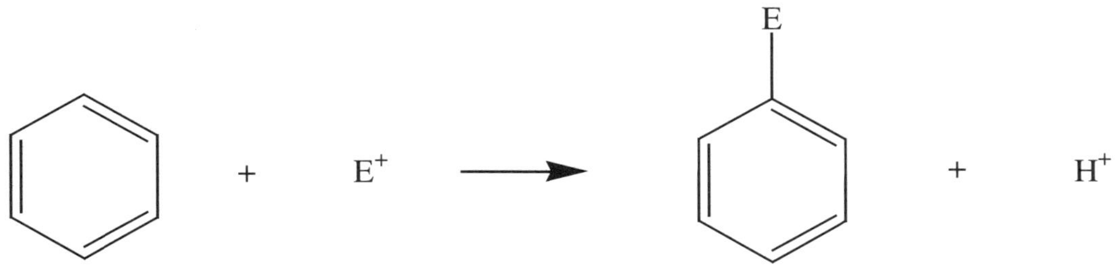

Electrophiles: **Br_2/FeBr$_3$, Cl_2/FeCl$_3$, I_2/H$_2$O$_2$, HNO$_3$/H$_2$SO$_4$, SO$_3$/H$_2$SO$_4$, *CH$_3$Cl/AlCl$_3$**

*Friedel-Crafts reaction (Other hydrocarbon attachments possible)

Example of a benzene reaction with an electrophile:

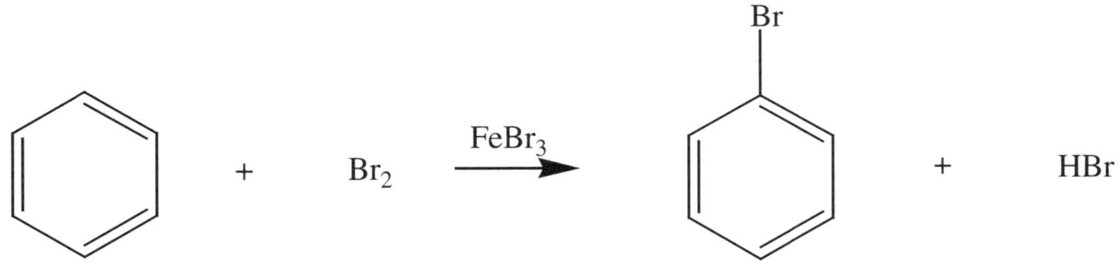

Positions on the benzene ring:

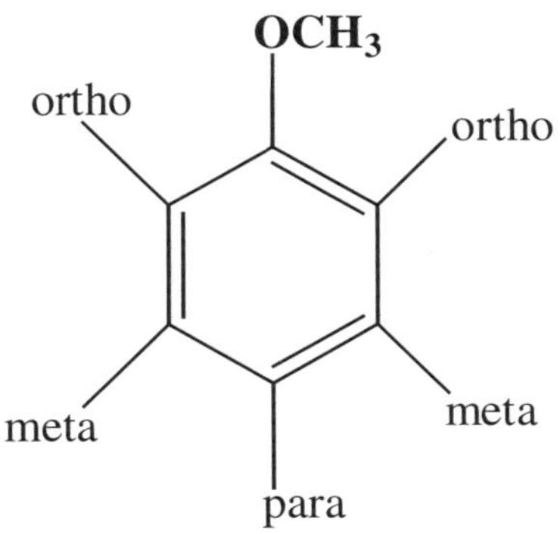

<u>Electrophilic addition with substituent in place:</u>

Activating group → ortho/para (with para placement first)

Activators (in order of strength): -NH$_2$, -NHR, -OH, -OCH$_3$, -C$_6$H$_5$, -CH$_3$

Deactivating group

Halogens (F, Cl, Br, I) →ortho/para (with para placement first)
Any other deactivator → meta
(Other deactivators: -NO$_2$, -CN, -COOH, -SO$_3$, -CHO)

<u>To help memorize:</u> (*General* rules)

Activators: (all *ortho/para* placement)
  Those with NH bound to something (either H or R group)
  Those with single-bond oxygen bound to something (either H or R group)
  Pure hydrocarbons (benzene, methyl, etc.)

Deactivators:

Halogens (F, Cl, Br, I) → special group of deactivators
All other deactivators include molecules with either:
  Double-bonded oxygen (NO$_2$, COOH, SO$_3$, CHO)
  Double-bonded nitrogen (CN)

<u>Memory tip:</u> All are placed in the para/ortho positions (activators and halogen deactivators) except for "double-bonded" deactivators. These "*mega*" bonds are added in the *meta* position.

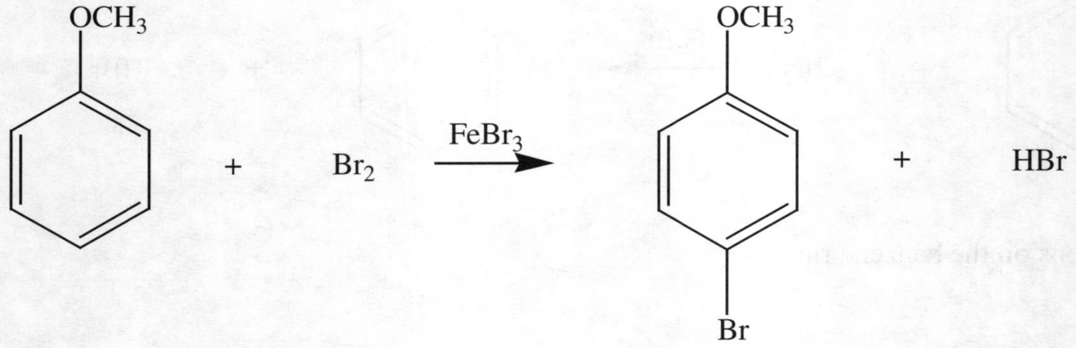

Activator : placed in para position

Activators (2): placement in ortho position

Deactivator (halogen): placement in para position

Deactivator (non-halogen): placement in meta position

OCH_3 + CH_3Cl $\xrightarrow{AlCl_3}$ product with OCH_3 (para) CH_3

Activator: electrophile to para position. (Friedel-Crafts alkylation)

2. Nucleophilic substitution may also occur in rare circumstance (extremely strong base)

Br, NO_2, NO_2, NO_2 + ^-OH $\xrightarrow{H_3O^+}$ OH, NO_2, NO_2, NO_2

Nucleophilic substitution of –OH for Br.

INFRARED SPECTROSCOPY

-OH	3,300-3,600	Strong, broad
-C=O	1,600	Strong, sharp
C-O-C	2,700	

Stability Facts

1. Heat of combustion (amount of energy released when carbon burnt with oxygen)
    Less energy released → *lower heat of combustion* → *more stable* the compound.
    More energy released → *higher heat of combustion* → *less stable* the compound.
2. In cyclohexane: a) *equatorial* is *more stable* than *axial.*
                       b) *chair conformation* is *more stable* than *boat.*
3. Carbocation: 3° (tertiary) more stable than 2° (secondary) more stable than 1°
                      (primary)
4. Free radicals: 3° is more stable than 2° is more stable than 1°.
5. In alkenes: *Trans* is more stable than *cis.*
                      Anti is more stable than *gauche.*
                      More substituted alkene → *more stable* → *lower the heat of
                      hydrogenation*
                      Less substituted alkene → *less stable* → *higher the heat of
                      hydrogenation*
6. Cyclic compounds: Less ring strain → more stable (cyclohexane *most* stable)

PHYSICS BOTTOM LINE

UNITS AND GEOMETRY

Circumference of a circle

Circ = $2\pi r$

Area of a sphere

A = πr^2

Surface Area of a sphere

A = $4\pi r^2$

Volume of a sphere

V = $\frac{4}{3}\pi r^3$

Pythagorean Theorem

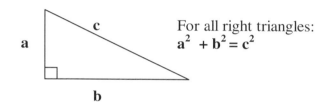

For all right triangles:
$a^2 + b^2 = c^2$

Trigonometric Functions

$\sin = \,^{\text{opposite}}/_{\text{hypotenuse}}$ **Hint**: "SOH"

$\cos = \,^{\text{adjacent}}/_{\text{hypotenuse}}$ "CAH"

$\tan = \,^{\text{opposite}}/_{\text{adjacent}}$ "TOA"

*Opposite and adjacent refer to lengths of the sides in relation to the angle.

Exponential Functions

■ **Multiplication**

$10^a + 10^b = 10^{a+b}$

$\log(ab) = \log a + \log b$

■ **Division**

$10^a / 10^b = 10^{a-b}$

$\log(^a/_b) = \log a - \log b$

VECTORS

Components

$a_x = a \cos \theta \qquad a_y = a \sin \theta$

Magnitude

$|a| = (a_x^2 + a_y^2)^{1/2}$

MOTION

Δ = "final minus initial"   OR   **Displacement**

$\Delta = x_f - x_i$

Average Velocity

$v_{av} = \Delta x / \Delta t$

Average Acceleration

$a_{av} = \Delta v / \Delta t$

Kinematics Equations

- $x_f = x_0 + v_0 t + \frac{1}{2} a t^2$
- $v_f = v_0 + at$
- $v_f^2 - v_0^2 = 2a\Delta x$

Relative Motion

$V_{pa} = V_{pb} + V_{ba}$

Centripetal Acceleration

$a_c = v^2/r$

Centripetal Force

$F_c = ma_c = mv^2/r$

FORCES

Weight	Friction	Newton's 2nd Law	Hooke's Law (spring force)
$W = mg$	$F = \mu N$	$F = ma$	$F = -kx$

WORK AND POWER

Work (constant force)

$W = F \bullet d = F\, d \cos \theta$

Work and Kinetic Energy

$W_{net} = K_f - K_i = \Delta K$

Average Power

$P_{av} = W / \Delta t$

ENERGY AND MOMENTUM CONSERVATION

Kinetic Energy	Gravitational Potential (constant g)	Elastic Potential (spring)	Mechanical Energy
$KE = \frac{1}{2}mv^2$	$U_{grav} = mgh$	$U_{elas} = \frac{1}{2}kx^2$	$Mech = KE + U_{grav} + U_{elas}$

Momentum

$p = mv$

Impulse

$J = \Delta p = F\Delta t$

Work Done by Friction

$W_{nc} = -F_f d$

Center of Mass

$x_{cm} = \frac{1}{M} \sum m_i x_i$

ROTATION

- **Angular Displacement** $\Delta\theta = \theta_f - \theta_I$
- **Angular Velocity** $\omega = \frac{\Delta\theta}{\Delta t} = \frac{v}{r}$
- **Angular Acceleration** $\alpha = \frac{\Delta\omega}{\Delta t} = \frac{a}{r}$

Rotational Inertia (particle)	Angular Momentum	Torque	Rotational Kinetic Energy
$I = mr^2$	$L = I\omega$	$\tau = I\alpha = r F \sin\theta$	$KE_{rot} = \frac{1}{2} I \omega^2$

GRAVITATION

Law of Gravitation

$F = Gm_1m_2 / r^2$

Acceleration (g) (nonconstant g)

$g = GM/r^2$

Gravitation Potential

$U(r) = \frac{-GMm}{r}$

OSCILLATIONS

Frequency

$f = \frac{1}{T}$

Pendulum Period

$T = 2\pi \left(\frac{L}{g}\right)^{1/2}$

WAVES

- **Sinusoidal Position**
  $x(t) = x_m \cos(\omega t + \phi)$
- **Angular Frequency**
  $\omega = {}^{2\pi}/_T = 2\pi f$
  $\omega = ({}^k/_m)^{1/2}$ $({}^{spring}/_{mass})$
- **Traveling Wave Position**
  $y(x,t) = y_m \sin(kx - \omega t + \phi)$
- **Wave Velocity**
  $v = {}^\lambda/_T = f\lambda$

- **Beats**
  Number of beats $= f_{high} - f_{low}$
- **Sound Intensity**
  $\beta = 10dB \log(I/I_o)$
- **Doppler Effect**
  $f^l = (v \pm v_D) / (v \pm v_S)$

ELECTROMAGNETIC WAVES

Speed of Light

$c = f\lambda = 3.8 \, {}^m/_s$ in a vacuum

GEOMETRICAL OPTICS

Law of Reflection	$\theta_i = \theta_r$
Snell's Law (refraction)	$n_1 \sin\theta_1 = n_2 \sin\theta_2$
Index of Refraction	$n = c_{vacuum} / c_{medium}$
Internal Reflection	$\sin\theta_c = n_2/n_1$
Focal Length of Mirror	$f = {}^R/_2$
Image/Object Relation	$1/d_i + 1/d_o = {}^1/_f$
Magnification	$m = -d_i/d_o = h_i/h_o$
Simple Magnifier	$m \sim 15 \, {}^{cm}/_f$

WAVE OPTICS

Interference Maxima

$d \sin\theta = m\lambda$ $(m = 0,1,2...)$

THERMODYNAMICS

Thermal Expansion	$\Delta L = L\, \alpha\, \Delta T$
Heat Capacity (C)	$Q = C\,(T_f - T_i)$
Specific Heat (c)	$Q = cm\,(T_f - T_i)$
Heat of Transformation (L)	$Q = Lm$
Conduction	$H = {}^{Q}\!/_{T}$ $= kA\,(T_H - T_C)/L$
1st Law of Thermodynamics	$\Delta E = Q + W$ $= Q - P\Delta V$
Efficiency (work or power)	x_{output}/x_{input}

FLUIDS

- **Density**
  $\rho = {}^{m}\!/_{V}$
- **Pressure**
  $P = {}^{\Delta F}\!/_{\Delta A}$
- **Pascal's Principle**
  $F_1/A_1 = F_2/A_2$
- **Lift**
  $lift = \Delta P * A$
- **Bernoulli's Equation**
  $p_1 + {}^{1}\!/_{2}\,\rho v_1{}^2 + \rho gh_1 = p_2 + {}^{1}\!/_{2}\,\rho v_2{}^2 + \rho gh_2$

- **Specific Gravity**
  $sg = \rho_{fluid}/\rho_{water}$
- **Hydrostatic Pressure**
  $p = p_o + \rho gh$
- **Equation of Continuity**
  $R = Av = constant$
- **Buoyant Force**
  $F = W_{disp} = \rho V_{disp} g$

ELECTROSTATICS

Coulomb's Law	Electric Field	Charge in Electric Field	Flux	Electric Potential	Point Charge Potential
$F = kq_1q_2/r^2$	$E = F/q_o$	$F = qE$	$\Phi_E = E \cdot A$ $\Phi_B = B \cdot A$	$V = U/q_o$ $\Delta V = \Delta U/q_o$	$V_{pt\ chg} = {kq}/{r}$

ELECTRICAL CIRCUITS

- **Capacitance**
  $C = {Q}/{V}$
- **Parallel Capacitors**
  $C_{eq} = C_1 + C_2$
- **Dielectric Constant (κ)**
  $C^1 = \kappa C$
- **Series Resistors**
  $R_{eq} = R1 + R2$
- **Power in Resistor**
  $P = i^2R = VI = V^2/R$
- **Power of Battery**
  $P = \varepsilon I$
- **AC Voltage**
  $\varepsilon = \varepsilon_o \sin(\omega t)$

- **Series Capacitors**
  $1/C_{eq} = (1/C_1 + 1/C_2)$
- **Energy in Capacitors**
  $U = {}^1\!/_2\ CV^2$
- **Ohm's Law**
  $V = IR$
- **Parallel Resistors**
  $1/R_{eq} = 1/R_1 + 1/R_2$
- **Resistivity**
  $R = {\rho L}/{A}$
- **RC Circuit (discharge)**
  $i = i_o e^{-t/RC}$
- **Average AC Power**
  $P_{av} = i^2_{rms}R = {}^1\!/_2\ P_{max}$

MAGNETIC FIELDS

Lorentz Force
$F = qv \times B$
$F = iL \times B$

QUANTUM PHYSICS

Photon Energy	Photon Momentum	Photoelectric Effect	Hydrogen Atom Energy Levels
$E = hf$	$p = h/\lambda$	$hf = \varphi + KE$	$E = -13.6 \text{ eV}/n^2$

NUCLEAR PHYSICS

Radioactive Decay

$$R = R_o e^{-\lambda t}$$
$$N = N_o e^{-\lambda t}$$

Half Life

$$t_{1/2} = \frac{\ln 2}{\lambda}$$

Mass-Energy Conversion

$$\Delta E = \Delta mc^2$$

$$t_{1/2} = {}^{\ln 2}/_{\lambda}$$

Mass-Energy Conversion

$$\Delta E = \Delta m c^2$$